My Fifty Years in Nursing

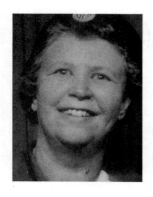 **Doris R. Schwartz, RN, MS, FAAN,** received her diploma in nursing from Methodist Hospital in Brooklyn, and bachelor's and master's degrees from New York University. During a 50-year career in nursing, she practiced public health nursing in many different places and taught public health nursing at Cornell University—New York Hospital School of Nursing. After retiring in 1980, she spent 10 years as Senior Fellow at the School of Nursing, University of Pennsylvania. Ms. Schwartz was a founding Fellow of the American Academy of Nursing, the first nurse to receive a Fogarty Fellowship for study of geriatric care in Scotland, and a member of the World Health Organization's Expert Committee on Nursing.

She has authored or co-authored numerous journal articles and books. As an early nursing author, she wrote, with Dr. Walter Modell, *Handbook of Cardiology in Nursing*, published by Springer Publishing Company in 1952 and reissued in four editions. Other books by her include *The Elderly Chronically Ill Patient* and *Geriatrics and Geriatric Nursing*, which won an AJN Book-of-the-Year Award. An earlier version of her present book, then titled *Give Us To Go Blithely: My Fifty Years of Nursing*, also won an AJN Book-of-the-Year Award in 1991.

MY FIFTY YEARS *in* NURSING

Give Us
To Go Blithely

Doris R. Schwartz, RN, MS, FAAN

SPRINGER PUBLISHING COMPANY

A previous edition of this book was published in 1990 by the author as *Give Us to Go Blithely: My Fifty Years of Nursing.*

Springer Publishing Company, Inc.
536 Broadway
New York, NY 10012-3955

Cover and interior design by Tom Yabut
Production Editor: Pamela Ritzer

95 96 97 98 99 / 5 4 3 2 1

Library of Congress Cataloging in Publication Data

Schwartz, Doris R.
　My fifty years in nursing : give us to go blithely / Doris Schwartz.
　p. cm.
　Includes bibliographical references and index.
　ISBN 0-8261-8920-2
　1. Schwartz, Doris R.　2. Nurses—United States—Biography.
　3. Public health nurses—United States—Biography.　4. Nursing.
　5. Schwartz, Doris R.
　[DNLM: 1. Nurses—personal narratives. 2. Nursing—personal narratives.
WZ 100 S3995 1995]
　RT37.S38A3　1995
　610.73'092—dc20
　[B]
　DNLM/DLC
　for Library of Congress　　　　　　　　　　　　　　94-24237
　　　　　　　　　　　　　　　　　　　　　　　　　　　　　CIP

Printed in the United States of America

Portions of this book have previously appeared in somewhat different form in the following publications: *The New York Times Sunday Magazine, The Reader's Digest, The Catholic World, Yankee Magazine, American Journal of Nursing.* Permission has been granted for the use of this copyrighted material. The courtesy of the publishers of these publications is gratefully acknowledged.

Contents

Preface

This compilation of memories was completed on my 75th birthday, ten years after I suffered from a serious stroke and retired from a fifty-year career in nursing. Some of the book's content has been stored solely in my mind, while much of it has come from a journal kept throughout the past fifty years.

Re-reading this book brings back memories of a deeply satisfying career, adventurous and crowded with friendships and travel to many parts of the world. Primarily my work has been concentrated in New York City, my birthplace, and at the New York Hospital-Cornell University Medical Center, where I worked for twenty-nine years. Many of the people and places described were encountered through outreach programs of that Center and its schools. Other events related to educational experiences undertaken by me in order to accept more senior responsibilities at Cornell.

When I first entered a hospital nursing school in September of 1939, we all believed that health care technology was thoroughly advanced. Yet by comparison with today's standards, hospital equipment was almost primitive. No Central Supply department existed, and disposable products were all but unknown. Packaged materials were being sterilized for the entire hospital at night in the operating room. Syringes and needles for hypodermic injections were boiled in the nursing units just before their use. The needles had to be individually hand-sharpened.

Back then a pre-operative hypodermic to produce sedation was prepared by boiling water in a tablespoon, the handle of which had been bent around an alcohol lamp. You learned to dissolve a small chalky tablet of the appropriate drug in the boiling water, drew the preparation into the newly-boiled syringe, then added the needle. Talking supportively to the patient, you assured him that he would return to the ward still anesthetized—Recovery Rooms not having been invented. You injected the morphine and scopolamine and explained that you would be right there when the patient woke up.

Antibiotics were still unknown. We depended on "sterile technique" and hand-washing to keep infection from spreading. Blood transfusions were relatively infrequent and still, at times, required the donor to be physically present. As the sulfa drugs came into existence, they were rightly called "miracle drugs." I administered penicillin for the very first time while in the Army during World War II. It was still an unstable solution, requiring that every dose be mixed just before injection from a powdered form and sterile water, and it had to be administered every three hours.

While the technology of nursing has undergone a revolution in the past fifty years, some of my best lessons in how to nurse were my earliest ones. I remember vividly the first dying old person I ever cared for when I was a student nurse. It was a learning experience and stayed with me for half a century.

I was giving morning care to a feverish, dehydrated, dry-skinned old man, under the supervision of an instructor with outstanding clinical skills. As I rubbed the patient's skin with oil, I heard him say, "How did you know that could feel so good?" Later he added, "Why didn't someone do that sooner?" My instructor told me to stay with the patient. He was tugging at the bed clothes restlessly. He was going to die very soon. The instructor told me the patient needed to know that someone cared for him. He had no family to send for.

That old man taught me a great deal in his last sixty minutes of life as I sat by his bedside. Sometimes we talked, briefly and quietly. Sometimes we were just there together, not speaking yet sensing our togetherness. I learned a valuable lesson that caring *about* a patient can be as important as providing care *for* the patient. Occasionally I am asked whether old people are afraid of death. That has not been my observation as a geriatric nurse. What many old people fear, it seems to me, is the thought of dying without being missed, of dying without one's absence mattering to anyone.

* * * *

My parents were hard-working, thrifty people. In our home money was not easily come by and it was saved or spent thoughtfully and generally with wisdom.

From an early age I received a weekly allowance. It began with a nickel, grew as I grew, to a dime, a quarter, and in high school I think it was a dollar. Whatever the amount there was a formula which guided its use. A portion (known as a tithe) went in one's Sunday School envelope ("for others"), a portion went into the piggy bank (against "hard times"). Pennies, and later larger coins, might buy a pencil, a pad, an eraser, a ball, a birthday gift for a friend, or sometimes a personal luxury of a Cracker Jack box with a prize in it, a Saturday (silent) movie or a trolley-car trip to Coney Island.

Against this rather puritanical approach to lavish spending, my father introduced a joyous custom known as "cherry money." He was a manufacturer and retailer of baskets. Baskets, in the first quarter of this century, were a luxury item. Filled with hothouse flowers, preserves, or luscious fresh fruit, they were known as "Streamer Baskets," delivered as a Bon Voyage gift to a passenger on an ocean-going liner, or to a private home in celebration of a holiday.

During the few weeks of the year when fresh cherries were in season (remember, this was in a pre-airplane, pre-delivery truck, pre-electric refrigeration era), fruit peddlers sold cherries in bulk and the city was hungry for them. My father then undertook a "second business." We would call it "moonlighting" today. He cleared out surplus wood and basket splints from the factory by cutting uncovered round wooden bases and surrounding them with woven tag ends of basket splits to make an unusual package which could hold a single layer of oversized, shining cherries, their burnished beauty gleaming beneath a piece of transparent waxed paper, held in place with a twist of string. Oh, how those beautifully packaged cherries sold!

At the close of the six-week cherry season he always brought the "cherry money" home, in cash. By definition, "cherry money" was exempt from all the rules of responsible spending. "Cherry money" didn't have to be accounted for. One was almost encouraged to be outrageously spendthrift with it, using it for something one wanted immensely but could never, in good conscience, buy.

My mother would buy an incredibly foolish hat, of chiffon and of an enormous size. My father bought opera tickets for her and himself. My brother and I were likely to obtain such longed-for items as a baseball bat, a pair of roller skates, and, the year I was seven, "cherry money" bought my first watch—an Ingersoll with figures that glowed in the dark. Oh, the sheer delight of that annual spending spree!

The joy of "cherry money" has always remained. My father died when I was eleven. Adolescence and early adulthood in the years of the great Depression were not easy. By the age of sixteen I was working steady (and for little pay). But always, by a burst of effort, there were "now and then" ways of earning small amounts of extra money. This I knew as "cherry money," to be accounted for separately, divided with others, and treated as a bonanza.

In fifty years of work as a nurse, I used money responsibly. But from time to time I earned small sums from writing about nursing. Every cent of money earned from writing went into a "cherry money" fund. One of the great joys of my adult life, the long-term foster parenting of three families of children, has been funded through my "cherry money." Another joyous experience, owning a former one-room rural schoolhouse in the foothills of the Pocono Mountains, was made possible through "cherry money."

Today, through the foster children of three "cherry money" families, I am foster grandparent to an Asian (Korean) grand-daughter, and Hispanic (Colombian) grandson, and American black boys and girls. Nothing in life has been a greater source of happiness than these foster families, now grown, with whom I am still in touch.

This book is another kind of "cherry money," one of the bonan-zas of being a nurse. Since 1939 there has been a continuous stream of work with people, in and from many lands. Nursing has given me joy in the way that my parent's concept of "cherry money" gave me joy. I have written for the nursing profession for many years, text books and professional articles.

But the stories of people contained herein, stored in diaries or in the corner of my memory, are like scraps of wood and bits of bas-ket splits in my father's factory, too colorful and useful to waste, though they are not the contents of traditional literature. They are a kind of human "cherry money," a human bonanza to be used to bring joy.

And so, retirement, with more free time available, the memorable adventures, the patients, the colleagues of fifty years in nursing, have recreated themselves into this human "cherry money" of a lifetime, to tell the story of one individual's nursing experiences, to present a verbal "slide show" that has given me gifts beyond my wildest imagination as a student.

Best of all, any proceeds that may be derived from this book will go to the University of Pennsylvania's School of Nursing, in order that future nurses may be helped to prepare for great adventures of their own in the world of the 21st Century.

The reader might wonder why I chose the subtitle I did for this book. It comes from the writings of Robert Louis Stevenson during his exile in Samoa. The paragraph from which it is taken sums up my own feelings about my life's journey:

> "The day returns and brings us the pretty round of irritating concerns and duties....Help us to perform them with laughter and kind faces. Let cheerfulness abound with industry. Give us to go blithely on our business all this day. Bring us to our resting beds weary and content and undishonored and grant is in the end the gift of sleep."

I can think of no better wish for a nurse about to begin a career of service to others.

Chapter 1

From Where You Are To Where You Need To Be

January 14, 1979. I woke at about 5:30 a.m. Something was wrong. It wasn't that I was sick, although I did feel light-headed. But like the old lady on the King's Highway in that long-ago nursery rhyme: "Lack-a-mercy on me, this is never I."

The room was very dark. I had no idea what time it was. The dial of the clock was lighted, but the face, appeared to be missing. I reached for the, light switch, but misplaced my hand in groping for the familiar spot. It wasn't there! I reached again and again but I couldn't find it.

I tried to get out of the bed but the wave of light-headedness washed in again. I was going to fall and wondered, "is this a drug reaction?" I was newly on Insulin and Dilantin. But I'd never had a drug reaction before. "No, it can't be that. I'd be shaky and have a rapid heartbeat. I'd be sweating. It must be a T.I.A. Or an aborted 'drop attack.' I'm wide awake, but I'd have fallen if I hadn't been sitting on the bed.

"Where's the clock? I can see the light on it. Where is the light switch? Not where it should be. Oh" that's what's wrong! I can't see! My God, I've been incontinent! I'll have to get help.

"I'm blind! It's getting lighter outside but I can't see anything in the room. I'm not really blind. The sun is starting to rise. I can't focus. Maybe if I rest quietly this will go away."

It didn't go away. It was a completed stroke.

Being adult, being in charge of oneself, means being able to get from where you are to where you need to be. Who said that? (I think it was Ambassador John Winant, referring to, President Franklin Roosevelt's disability.) Not focusing visually and not being able to bear weight was a double burden. It seemed to cut out all possibility of creative planning for the final eighteen months of work before I was scheduled to retire. They had done me the honor, in my sixty-fourth year, to promote me to a clinical associate professorship of public health nursing in the Cornell Medical College.

I remember the terrible chagrin at myself, "the uncooperative patient," the whole list of scares. "Am I going to lose my job?" And later, "Am I going to recover my vision? Can I finish this book? Will I ever be able to sleep through the night again?"

With this double disability—unless I got on top of it—there was no way I could return to clinical teaching. I had to tackle and succeed at one more piece of teaching, or patient-care demonstration in geriatric nursing, before I retired, and after that I would still have a lot of living to do.

In the end, I realized I was not so totally depressed with this spell of illness. This was enormously better than my first hospitalization the year before. Maybe I had finally learned how to be a patient. In any event it stopped being a nightmare, but for a long while I still couldn't clearly see my way out of it. Reality had validated the nightmare. Hopefully, I felt that reality would validate the escape plan—when I designed an escape plan.

Because I was a good rehabilitation nurse, I knew what had to be done. Daily swimming and nightly use of a stationary bicycle improved my balance and walking and I moved from a walker to a four-point cane to an ordinary one, while walking both faster and further. I learned to refocus my vision. A course in Orientation and Mobility Training was a great help with vision-related mobility problems. Others helped me and I helped myself. Long, long before I was a patient, I was a nurse.

Did I always want to be a nurse? Perhaps not always. As a child, I was fascinated by two other trades. Sailors, it seemed to me, were the luckiest people in the world. To live aboard a ship, to travel, to speak with personal knowledge of strange lands—that was the perfect life. I wanted to be a sailor but I was told, "Girls can't." It sounded stupid but there was no arguing with adults in the 1920s. They always won.

The other calling I looked on with envy was that of the man who read the gas meters on our block. What a job he had! Fuller Brush men, insurance agents, even peddlers, with their fine mysterious wares, were turned away from many doors, but the man who read the gas meters got into every house.

To get into people's houses and discover how they lived seemed to me, at the age of ten, more exciting than anything else. Adults, always discouraging, assured me that I could not become a reader of gas meters. "Girls don't go into strangers' homes like that."

So I became a nurse. In that capacity I sailed the Pacific on a war-time hospital ship. I visited foreign lands and spoke with personal knowledge of a wide assortment of colorful, friendly people.

As a visiting nurse, I climbed unknown house steps, rang unknown bells, and was welcomed into other people's homes in a New York tenement district, all day long.

Sometimes adults are not so smart. They don't know that in nursing you find the adventure of caring for people. A colleague of mine in the World Health Organization was nursing consultant to Outer Mongolia. Imagine that!

Prior to World War II and for several years directly after leaving the Army Nurse Corps, I worked in the Red Hook district, as a staff nurse, with the Visiting Nurse Association of Brooklyn, one of the oldest agencies of its kind in the nation. It was known as a training ground for public health nurses, absorbing large numbers of students and young graduates into a first experience in community health work.

This innovative, non-profit agency combined a portion of its nursing staff with that of the New York City Health Department to undertake a classic demonstration known as the Red Hook Experiment. It was one of the first combined-service agencies in which each nurse became the primary public health nursing-care provider to a small, overcrowded district.

Each acted as visiting nurse, school nurse and, on certain days of the week, nurse in that district's Child Health Station. Shopkeepers, school children, janitors and dock workers all had a genuine feeling of friendliness for their public health nurse and the feeling was mutual. A large center-city took on the human aspects of a village in the plan of the Red Hook Experiment.

My district along the Brooklyn waterfront is an area which would make a perfect background for a moving picture, a wonderful, colorful, comic, tragic spot, with blocks of rundown houses reflecting bits of many cultures: Syrian, Greek, Italian, Puerto Rican, American Indian among them. Churches, customs, and traditions of half a dozen different lands are to be found along a single street.

One of the constantly recurring surprises is the discovery that from many of these tenements along the harbor the kitchen window's view of the Statue of Liberty is as fine as from any of the high-rent buildings in the city. One day, just at sunset, in a room up five creaky flights of stairs, I turned from boiling a syringe to see a sky of flaming reds and purples. A crippled old Italian workman, whose life had been very hard, sat in his chair and watched the colors changing. He pointed to a brightly-tinted picture of his patron saint, then turned back to the window where Liberty was bathed in sunset.

"It's good," he said. "That saint from the old country, this one from New York. Both saints take care of me. You too?"

February 19, 1948. You get to know so many different kinds of people in this job. Take Dick, for instance. Dick is fourteen and with luck he would have started high school in September. Instead, at the end of August he broke his neck diving into shallow water. Thirty-nine days on the hospital's critical list brought him to a state of "hopeful paraplegia," in which sensation gradually came back to a body totally paralyzed from the neck down.

Dick came home to a basement apartment where his family of eight (five children younger than he) lives on a mighty limited income. There, the nurse turns up each day to help him exercise, to teach his mother how to put him in his braces, to supervise the whole round-the-clock plan of rehabilitation between his visits to the hospital clinic, which will one day send him back to school able to walk and use his hands again.

His mother needs a lot of help with other problems. The three-year-old is resenting all the time she spends with Dick and is behaving the way a three-year-old often does when a new baby replaces him in the family. Dick's mother, recovering from a serious illness of her own, and worn out by the strain and worry over her injured son, is just too troubled to take things calmly. She needs to talk about the pressures of bringing Dick through his siege and helping him to be a normal, well-adjusted adolescent.

March 12. Sometimes a chance remark makes more friends than all one's carefully-planned health teaching. I made a visit to a recently-arrived Italian family. Only the daughter could speak English:

"Yes, Papa and Tony have work as cabinetmakers. Yes, Mama liked the American hospital—first time she had ever been in a hospital for a baby. But she couldn't eat the American food. Yes, she understands all about the baby, thank you. She has brought up seven. The baby's name is going to be 'America'."

This family, though new, is quite self-sufficient. They have a family doctor. A couple of minutes to acquaint them with the community resources and the visiting nurses' services, a check to see that the pre-school children have completed their immunizations, and a cordial farewell all around. "Please tell your mother that I hope she and all the family will be very happy in America."

A quick translation and an emotional outburst of Italian. "Mama says, thank you. You are the first person, not Italian, to tell her I hope you are happy here."

Times like that I wish I could speak Italian. Even more often I wish I could speak Spanish so I could really talk with my many Puerto Rican families. Schoolchildren act as interpreters for some things, but you can't go into a home and ask a child to tell his mother why his father has to come to the syphilis clinic. It is also very hard to have a mother ask for birth control information through her small child, particularly if the family is Catholic.

If there are no school children, the language barrier is formidable. A Greek seaman who was a newly diagnosed diabetic, and would be on his ship in three days, was responsible for taking insulin. I had no Greek and he had no English. You can teach any skill by showing, but you need words to help someone understand the reason behind it. This new diabetic learned how to take insulin, and that's a fairly complex procedure, because he trusted me, but I couldn't teach him to change his diet without his understanding why and without my learning what his diet was. And it seems too bad to have the enormous advantage of sitting at a Puerto Rican woman's table, in an attitude of mutual respect and friendliness, and not be able to convey ideas along with the technique of taking Junior's temperature.

I'd be glad to swap any number of college points in Philosophy of Education and History of Education for the ability to say in simple Spanish sentences, "Look, Mrs. Rodrigues, nobody on earth can give your baby the things you and your husband can. Your good sense, the feeling you have for him, and your belief in what he can become are the most important things he will ever have.

"The doctors and the nurses don't want you to think they know more than you do. They just want you to let them help with some of the problems you don't know how to handle; to show you why it is better to protect your baby by having him immunized and letting the doctor look him over now and then. The clinic is crowded sometimes and you have to wait and once in a while the people who work there get tired and irritable and they don't seem very friendly, but they really are your friends and your baby's friends.

"All the things that are worthwhile and important are a little hard to get. You know that, so if it seems like too much trouble to take the baby there, stop and remember how lucky you are to have the clinic to go to—how all your babies will have a chance to grow up well and strong instead of half of them dying the way you told me your mother's did, back in Puerto Rico twenty years ago."

But when I am looking up words in the dictionary one at a time and still have half-a-dozen home visits to make, I don't say that. I say, "Take him to the clinic, for sure. Nine o'clock, Thursday. And don't forget!" Even that means tuning a lot of pages in the well-worn pocket dictionary.

March 22. An old Syrian grandmother on Pacific Street has pneumonia. I was there on the verge of a religious holiday and at such times in the old country each village had the emblem of a different kind of cross baked into its bread. While I was taking care of my patient, I heard something being slapped down on the kitchen floor. Later, I looked in.

Newspapers were spread out on the floor and the women of the family were down on their knees with paddles, like small canoe paddles, bearing the emblem of their grandmother's village, slapping the design into each loaf of bread. The smell got nicer and nicer while I was finishing with grandmother. Before I went home, I had to accept a loaf of bread with the symbol on it; it showed that grandmother and I were in rapport.

April 8. I went to a Dean Street apartment to instruct a Mohawk Indian mother in the care of her daughter Beatrice's new eyeglasses. Because I am also Beatrice's school nurse, I was present at the child's eye examination in school. Then the prescription was made up by the Red Cross, and I was to bring it over.

Imagine my surprise to find a new Mohawk Indian family living there. What has happened to Beatrice? What should be done with the glasses? No one can help me. It is like Jerry Running Bear, a ten-year-old with a congenital clubfoot, who never arrived at the

Long Island College Hospital for his first operation. He is presumably back on the reservation on the Canadian border.

The Mohawks do high-steel construction. Sometimes an uncle and nephew come and form the backbone of a rivet gang, returning to the reservation far richer after several months of work in Manhattan. It is genetics that makes them able to sit on a narrow girder many stories up and catch a red-hot steel rivet with tongs, placing it where it belongs and, keeping their balance, catch the next rivet when it comes.

Perhaps the landlord does not even know that his tenants have changed—there is still a Mohawk family in the apartment and the rent is still being paid.

April 27. I visited after a home delivery today, arriving when Jose was all of two-and-a-half hours old. He was a pretty messy little boy since Papa, the only adult in sight, was occupied with the care of four other children, aged two to ten.

Home was a cold-water flat in a filthy building, but the apartment was neat and clean, although almost bare of furniture. Mama was in the only bed I saw, pleased as punch with her new son and with her own clever maneuvering to outwit the hospital system.

Apparently she had been told that if a doctor or a nurse caught you when you were pregnant, you had to go to a hospital. And a hospital, to this woman, was in every way a prison—an experience to be avoided at all costs.

So by not bringing the children to the Child Health Station, she managed to escape notice. Then, this morning, it was easy. She sent for the ambulance after instead of before the baby was born and escaped the hospital sentence.

I bathed Mama, whisking an occasional cockroach off the rim of the wash basin, and made her bed. An ancient neighbor woman volunteered her services at this point (mostly out of curiosity to see what was going on, I think). She obligingly washed out the bed linen and other odds and ends. Then, with Papa and the four boys looking on and making approving sounds in Spanish, I started to work on the baby.

The oldest boy spoke English. "I go to school here. Came from Puerto Rico this year," he informed me. "Papa makes $26 a week. Mama and Papa like having another boy. So do we. He can play ball with us some day. New York is better than Puerto Rico. We live good here."

I looked around the shabby apartment. "We live good here," and then I looked at the parents beaming proudly at each other and at those nice, relaxed, easy-to-live-with youngsters. Once again I wanted Spanish words to say the things I felt. Instead, I asked the boy, "How did you get enough money to come to New York?"

And the answer. "Papa was a G.I. Saved for the United States all the time he was in the Army. Much money then."

And Papa showed me his picture in uniform with corporal's stripes, Mama looking at the picture tenderly. She said something very softly and seriously in Spanish and the little boy said, "She says we—all the kids—should never have to be in a war. She would have *five* soldiers if we had to go to war."

And I wanted Spanish words again, but instead I rolled the baby up in a piece of blanket and pretended to bounce him down to her and everybody laughed when she held Jose in her arms and talked to him. We looked for a place for the baby to sleep, but there wasn't any.

We looked some more and found an old, cracked patent- leather suitcase. it was nice and roomy. So we stood two chairs together and put the suitcase on it and tied the lid back so that it couldn't close unexpectedly, and there was the nicest bed you could want for a fine new baby.

And everybody laughed again, and the boys all promised not to touch the baby or the suitcase unless their father was right there to show them how. Mother nursed the baby and when I left he was sound asleep in the well-worn suitcase, but he had every material thing a baby needed and a lot of love besides.

And I wished I could have told them less hesitantly that I thought Jose was a lucky baby and that for two cents I'd be willing to join them in that drafty, crowded flat. For you could always polish it up with soap and water and you could always flick the roaches off the washbowl, but you couldn't always, or even often, find a family that was such a close-knit unit.

For several days to come it will be fun to dash in there in the morning, and for several years to come there will be those five boys for the community nurses to keep an eye on, first in the Child Health clinic, then in the health room of the elementary school.

Maybe you can see now why I like this job. One day's assignment may include school nursing and bedside nursing in the home. Another day, time spent at the Child Health Station and some home visits; still another day may be spent in the clinic. It never gets monotonous. In fact, the Red Hook program would be fun to work in, forever.

Chapter 2

The Army Nurse Corps in World War II

Prior to, and during World War II, recruitment into military nursing was managed through the Red Cross Nursing Reserve Corps. As students, most of my classmates and I had joined the Corps, which was open to seniors in schools of nursing as well as to graduate nurses.

The Corps recruited for disaster work of all kinds, natural as well as man-made catastrophes. I think that few of us, when we signed up, really believed we would ever be involved in a global war. By the close of 1943, though, as the military services began to build up to more than 75,000 nurses, almost all of us found ourselves in uniform.

I was in the Army, and from the start, it felt like the Army. At that time basic training was not very different for health professionals than it was for the military. We trained under live ammunition; we marched and dug foxholes. But all this was out on Long Island, a pretty safe place to be.

For my whole career in the Army patients were moving back and forth, seemingly under my hands. This was certainly true during my first assignment, the Air Evacuation Center at Mitchel Field, Long Island, a rapidly-built barracks hospital where newly wounded soldiers were flown from Europe, to be sorted and given temporary treatment. It was a holding station; every day several hundred men would come in and several hundred would be flown out to major Army hospitals closer to their homes.

I was head nurse on an amputee ward. The patients were badly injured, but young and otherwise healthy. Many had been exposed to the war for so little time that it was almost a dream to them. There was an atmosphere of excitement—they were home in the United States again.

Add to that the fact that many things were being done, not only for their health, but for their comfort. The morale was high, and newspaper reporters and veterans organizations began to take notice and visit. It was quite a dynamic place to be, something like Grand Central Station but with everybody critically ill.

And from the moment their injured soldiers were back at Mitchel Field, the families too came tearing out to Long Island. They were told not to, that the men wouldn't be there for more than a few days and would be sent on to hospitals closer to home.

But they didn't wait. They showed up twenty-four hours a day. It was a very dramatic, emotional time. Men were seeing their new babies for the first time. Couples were breaking up right before your eyes, and parents were breaking down. Many felt their sons' lives were finished—you tried very hard to keep them from upsetting the open ward full of men in the same situation as their son.

Every morning you fed breakfast to fifty patients, got their papers and records together, gave them whatever medications they needed for the plane trip, got them loaded onto stretchers and into airplanes to all parts of the country. And very often the new batch landed before the last ones took off. You had patients on the beds, and patients on stretchers under the beds, or waiting on the floor for the beds to be newly made-up.

Later, I was stationed on the Army Hospital Ship *Marigold* in the Pacific theater. We treated the men coming out of Japanese prison camps, the men from Corregidor or Bataan. They had spent most of the war there, watching incredible numbers of fellow soldiers die of neglect. They were starving and demoralized.

There were about fifty of us—nurses, doctors and dentists (who did a lot of plastic surgery). We had periods of great activity and then, after we had delivered our patients back to the Philippines for more extensive treatment, week-long periods of relative calm as we went back for more patients.

In the Pacific, many harbors—Manila Bay, Okinawa, and Tokyo Bay—were known to be mined. The ship had to drop anchor at the mouth of the harbor, and patients would be brought out on flat-tops, barges that wouldn't hit a mine but just scoot over them. That meant boarding patients at sea, which was very hard. They had to be loaded onto stretchers and brought up with cranes. Sometimes we lifted as many as 775 in a 24-hour period, more exhausting for the patient than for us. He must have felt as if he had one chance in a hundred of not going down.

On my last assignment, at the great Army rehabilitation center known as Percy Jones General Hospital in Battle Creek, Michigan, I worked with individuals whom I finally was able to know on a long-term basis. It was not unusual for a patient there to have gone through a series of forty operations, over a period of several years.

There was a great deal of depression among the men, and not unexpectedly. The patient, for one thing, was upset at seeing surgeon after surgeon whom he had trusted getting out—out of the Army, now that the war was over. He lost his nurses as well. Many of my colleagues and I saw at this time that nursing and medicine could do something other than save lives. After the war was over, many of us had decided to stay in, at least until some of the reparative work was done.

My journals from these three distinct periods of Army service still remind me of the human cost of war and of our need to find better ways to resolve conflicts between people and among nations.

The Air Evacuation Transport Center, Mitchel Field, N.Y.

November 3, 1943. This morning, as we walked from our quarters to the hospital, the ambulances started rolling in—long lines of them painted with red crosses—creeping at a snail's pace along the rough dirt road to avoid jouncing.

You are ready with an empty ward and watch them bring in the litters, forty-five at a time. You never know what is coming next. Yet you can always count on the next hectic thirty minutes being absolutely packed with an assortment of emotions such as one would ordinarily experience in a lifetime. Pain, humor, courage, happiness all appear at once and rather than merging, they stand out as a dozen or more clear distinct flashes, parading a whole story before you in an instant, then fading into the routine of a busy hospital ward.

You learn to size up situations quickly, almost intuitively. One part of you says coolly, "Put that next patient in Bed 3." You grin at him and say, "Hi, soldier, you sure must have worked at growing that beard." He looks pathetically small on the stretcher, and you realize suddenly that both his legs are gone.

The realization and the sharp stab of pain that it brings, and the grin and the kidding remark that you toss at him are all separate thoughts and emotions, yet all told, they do not occupy thirty seconds. Then you turn to the next stretcher and begin again.

They're dead tired, these G.I.s, and hot and dirty, but their tongues never stop. "Fresh milk! Hey, fellas, its COLD! Y'oughta taste Limey drinks; they dunno what iced means."

"Where are we now? Can we call our folks? Are there visitors allowed here?"

"Careful when you move me, lady. 'Taint that I'm fussy, but I fall apart easily."

"Boy, it's good to see American girls again, the kind you can sling a line to without having them believe you."

"Listen, beautiful, can we get a beer here? Huh, not even ONE? Hey, guys, no beer here. There must be a war on!"

Finally they're fed, bathed and settled comfortably. Then comes the inevitable, "Whaddya know about the amputation centers, nurse? Think they can fix me up as good as new? Will I be able to dance? Ride a motorcycle? Boy, will I impress the folks!" They're anxious, a little unsure, but confident of complete recovery.

Over in the corner, an older man, one pajama sleeve empty, sits looking into space. "That's fine with legs," he mutters to himself. "Artificial arms won't play pianos, though!"

I mentally pick him out for a lot of special attention, and later on discover how much harder it is for a brilliant and gifted individual like this to adjust than it is for the less-talented and less-educated soldiers with whom we deal more often. Odd, isn't it, that the more we have in this world, the more difficult it seems to come face to face with hard situations? You would almost expect it to be the other way around.

By noon, dressings are changed, broken casts replaced and life has settled down to a routine. The G.I.s have taken us completely in their stride and as the next planeload arrives and the ambulances pull up to the ward next door six hours later, they lean from the windows and call to the newcomers with all the wisdom of old timers, 'Whatta country club! They sure treat ya good, here. Brother, your days of wandering are over! Come in and find a home!" And in the next ward, the same thing is beginning all over again.

We had a brand new gang come in this afternoon, especially full of pep and exceptionally likable. One amputee, an incredible-looking youngster, brought with him the world's largest crop of freckles, a G.I. haircut of very red hair, and a voice that could be heard in San Francisco as he yodeled his sentiments on being back in the United States. He telephoned his home (in Wisconsin) from his bed, and the entire ward grinned contentedly to hear him shriek, "Hey, Mom! Mom! It's me!" I laughed too, but unaccountably I wanted to cry. He was so very young to be coming home, with two strikes against him for the rest of his life.

Most of the time (and always with the patients) I can be enthusiastic about the wonderful job the medics and the rehabilitation people are doing, but once in a while it catches up with me, the awful waste—of lives and potential happiness—and the terrific adjustments ahead, not just now, while they're young and good natured and heroes in the eyes of the public, but over the next sixty years when one by one they'll have to fight it out alone.

December 1, 1943. The nurses were very busy today: doctors' rounds, complicated dressings, demands of sick patients. It was almost ten o'clock when we got around to the back half of the ward. When we got there (it's where the less-seriously injured ones are put) all the patients had gotten up and, hopping around on their one leg, were making the beds and cleaning the place to help out.

They beamed like so many angelic choir boys and said pensively, "We didn't want to make any extra work when you were doing so much, so we figured we could get fixed up in here." I was prouder of those bumpy beds and that sketchily swept floor than I usually am of the ward's spotless appearance.

The group of wounded we have with us now are unusually appreciative of attention, the little comforts and luxuries we can give them. They're a noisy, cheerful lot, but their constant gaiety is forced—a shield to protect them from thinking too deeply. I was kidded by one of them about something last night and we were laughing together easily.

Suddenly his eye fell on a page of an old *Life* magazine which his buddy was glancing at. His whole body tensed. "See that picture," he said rapidly, "that's where I was hit. We passed that spot a couple of hours earlier. When I got it," he said a moment later, "there were only six guys in my whole company who hadn't been hit. Don't ever let anybody kid you, Nurse. When you're in it you don't pray that you won't get hit, you just pray that you'll be one of the ones that gets hit and lives instead of one who gets hit and don't."

I glanced around at the others who were listening. They looked years older than they had ten minutes ago.

"That's right," they agreed. "It's almost a relief when it comes." And, "You feel like hell leaving the other guys to take it, but something stronger than your mind tells you you've been lucky." The soldier who said that was nineteen years old and minus a leg.

May 29, 1944. Louis was an uncommonly apprehensive soul, even for a patient with a diagnosis of "combat fatigue." About 2 a.m. he appeared at the office, looking sleepy but worried.

"Lieutenant," he said politely, but in uncertain tones, "Could you do something about the goat under my bed?"

"The what?" I asked.

"Please," he repeated, "I think there's a goat under my bed."

None of my suggestions about shadows or dreams shook his certainty. "Would you feel better, Louis, if we flashed the light under your bed so that you can see for yourself that nothing is there?"

He thought that would be fine, so I took my flashlight and we crept softly into the ward, not to waken the others. Whispering a heartening, "See, Louis," I flashed the light under the bed.

Two large eyes under two long and well-formed horns peered out at us with interest and there was a distinctly goatish odor. As I stared, spellbound, the goat stretched out his neck and nonchalantly sampled my shoe laces.

Louis, with a faint sigh of relief, mumbled that he hadn't thought he "could go crazy that quick," and he flopped onto the bed and went to sleep, leaving me with a flashlight in one hand and a handful of goat fur in the other, in the darkened ward. We never did find out how the animal got into the hospital, though we suspected that he had been collected by some young officers returning from a party.

July 20. During his month of front-line combat one of our patients had picked up a German camera containing a roll of film which had been half used. He and his buddies shot the rest of the film and it was developed here at the hospital. There were four prints of our patient and his pals, grimy and bearded, and four prints of a blond German soldier of perhaps twenty-one with a towheaded baby on his lap and a wife gazing at him adoringly.

Our soldiers looked at the print a long time without speaking. A few weeks ago our entire ward had been theoretically out to exterminate that German and now they were wishing quietly that his wife had somehow got those pictures.

The patient who now owned the camera shuffled the pictures again. "I never saw my kid," he said softly. "He was born after I went over and he died a couple months later."

Slowly he tore up the German soldier's prints. And somebody turned on the radio, very loud.

September 11. We start to make rounds, rolling the dressing cart from bed to bed. The surgeon, a regular-army colonel, questions each new patient—so very kindly. "How long were you in combat?"

"One day, sir."

"Just a week."

A soldier from Georgia forces a matter-of-fact expression as he indicates his shattered feet. "Reckon they'll have to come off, don't you, sir?"

The surgeon doesn't answer for a moment and then puts his arm gently around the boy's shoulders.

"You knew that, didn't you?" he asks, and the boy nods violently and turns and smothers his sobs with a pillow.

"Why?" "Why?" "Why?"

Must every visiting family expect you to explain why it had to happen to *their* soldier? They look at you pleadingly, as though you could change the facts. They seem to hope against hope that you've mixed him up with somebody else in the ward.

You want to shout that it doesn't matter if you do mix them up, that every one of them is equally tragic and badly injured. But you say what wonderful work the rehabilitation centers are doing, and you give questioners some aromatic spirits and you tell a mother to be sure to tease her son about his G.I. haircut.

She clutches eagerly at the idea, for she wants to help make the next couple of minutes go smoothly. The other fellows know it's a hard time and they all help out: "Gee, Mom, you look just like your picture." "You know, you're kinda like my mom, too." "Bet Johnny gave those gray hairs to you. He sure gave them to our C.O." And suddenly they are all laughing and talking at once and you give a sigh of relief, for they don't need your help any more. You think, what great people they are, all of them.

Aboard the Army Hospital Ship *Marigold*

I was stationed on the Army hospital ship *Marigold* in Yokohama Harbor from shortly before V-J Day, September 2, through November 11, 1945. The *Marigold* was the very first American ship to enter Japanese home waters and it became the processing station for hundreds of Allied prisoners released from Japanese detention camps. Many of the American prisoners were regular Army veterans, as well as those who had volunteered or had been drafted once the war began.

Yokohama, September 2, V-J Day. This morning peace was signed aboard the *Missouri* in the outer harbor of the bay. The eyes of the whole world were on this spot, and landing barges poured wave after wave of troops ashore in never-ending lines.

Against this background, the officers and men of the *Marigold*, stretching their legs for the first time on Japanese soil, were busily engaged in a game of baseball. It was breathtaking and ironic. In the background world history was being made, and, in typically American fashion, our soldiers were playing sandlot baseball.

September 3. Today the first prisoners-of-war came aboard. There was none of the exuberance of the European P.O.W.s. These men were quiet and polite—almost apathetic about expressing themselves. There was no doubt about their joy and their appreciation of little things—cleanliness, fresh clothing, sheets, hot water. The showers were on continually; patient after patient emerged from them glowing, "God, that was good!"

The breeze blew a sprinkling of cigarette ashes across the whiteness of a bed sheet; instinctively, as the gray specks moved, a soldier reached to hit them. "Had lice for so long I take for granted that's what anything is that moves," he explained sheepishly.

September 4. Today they rolled up by the truckload—Americans, Australians, Dutch Colonials—veterans of a dozen different campaigns. It was hard to identify nationalities by uniforms, for their uniforms consisted of mixtures of all sorts, with a sprinkling of Navy, civilian, and Japanese clothing mixed in, patch on patch, until the most tattered American scarecrow seemed luxuriously dressed by comparison.

There were the usual incongruous notes: a ukulele lugged through three years of prison life by its determined possessor; Japanese flags and souvenirs. The warehouse on the dock was turned into a processing station, and the *Marigold* was permanently docked alongside. When the truckloads of liberated P.O.W.s arrived, they were taken to the warehouse, deloused and showered, issued clean clothing, and separated into the "unquestionably healthy" (who are well enough to return home via plane) and those who will need medical care for the trip.

The P.O.W.s to be admitted to the *Marigold* were carried aboard, and in an incredibly short time were lolling contentedly in our wards, enjoying the luxuries of cleanliness and security again. Yesterday's observations still held—they're a quiet crowd, quiet with the apathy born of long isolation and confinement.

I walked into a room ten minutes after the lunch trays were given out. A soldier wasn't eating. His tray had been brought without silver, and it simply hadn't occurred to that man to complain or ask for some. He was waiting till another patient finished, so he could use the silver from that tray. The predominating atmosphere on the ship tonight is weary satisfaction that the war is over.

September 5. It is such little things that make the strongest impressions on these men. White bread is "angel food." They lie awake at night because "the feel of a bed is so strange." No, they'd rather not have a sleeping pill, thank you. "It is so good to just lie here wide awake and know that you're free."

And still they talk with that same quiet politeness; even after a shot of penicillin they say, "Thank you."

There are a lot of beri beri cases; in fact, there are samples of every conceivable nutritional disease here. Many of the more apathetic individuals still seem unable to comprehend the full significance of their release. Others walk around the ship just looking, and touching objects as if to assure themselves of their reality.

A patient offers a cigarette to a wardman on deck. "I'd never have done that a week ago," he marvels.

Magazines—*Life,* the *Digest, Coronet,* the *Post*—all the old copies Special Services can produce are looked at eagerly. The date of the issue is of no importance: "Gotta see what America's like now."

They can't get over the miracle of being free of lice; for most, cleanliness heads all the list of things for which they are grateful. There are frequent arrivals with snow-white hair. One grizzled Navy man had not only white hair, but a full white beard. The tragedy of having to remove it was soul-shattering. He'd spent four years growing that beard, and if he could stand the lice, he didn't see why anyone else should be concerned.

When they talk about their life in the camps, the patients complain mainly of the lack of food, and the complete indifference of their captors to any of the considerations that are a part of our culture—fair play, humor, cooperation, courtesy—apparently not so much from a deliberate desire to infuriate and annoy the Americans, as from the fact that their behavior is standard for them. Many of the boys say the Japanese officers beat and kicked their own soldiers with as little regard as they displayed for Americans who provoked them.

Some of our arrivals today had worked (unwillingly) in Japanese industries. A soldier from Scotland said, "We worked 12 hours a day, and every fifth day we had to work 19 hours." Several added that the Japanese drove their own workers on schedules almost as rugged. They all agree, "You worked or you died." The food, scarce as it was, went only to those who produced. "If you produced enough they let you pretty much alone, but if you were sick or weak, or couldn't keep up with the rest, your game was up."

Men from many different camps estimated that fifteen to twenty percent of their number had died—usually from starvation, and usually in the early stages of the war. This at first seemed to refute their claim that the food became scarcer as the war continued, but their explanation was: "If you survived the first year, you were tough enough to want to stick it out. If you wanted to stick it out, you had to work harder than you ever worked before, sixteen to eighteen hours a day. After you'd done that for a year, you were too damn mad to die. We stole whatever food we could and carried it past the guards under our arms, in our underwear, in hats and shoes. If caught, it meant a severe beating—every man here has received more beatings than you could count on both hands."

September 6. The bunks already bear hometown signs. On the foot of one is "City Limits—Los Angeles." A soldier takes out a dog-eared snapshot of his family and shows it to you. It is the general signal for everyone to bring them out.

These tattered pictures were retained by great effort through the years, for the Japanese spitefully destroyed or marked up every personal possession they could find. The men tell you triumphantly how they saved them—in the straw ticking of a mattress, in the sole of a shoe—any device to keep that precious scrap of paper out of sight of their captors.

One soldier produced his souvenir bitterly. It was, I think, a tragic and ironic little happening of the war, though I'm sure it originated without malice. He had never once heard from his folks throughout all these years in prison camp. Hungry, sick, miserable, he lived for the day when just one letter would get through.

At Christmas last year his wish was granted. The envelope given him by the guards bore his name. He opened it eagerly. Inside was a gaily colored picture of a military party with wreaths, a lighted Christmas tree, and gifts in the background. Underneath were the words, 'We give thanks for the preservation of liberty and democracy in our land and we wish you well." It was signed, "The Mayor's Committee on Military Welfare" and came from the man's hometown.

"That," he said quietly, "was harder to take than the treatment of the Japanese."

September 7. The other hospital ships have come in to shore— the *Marigold* opposite the warehouse, the Dutch one at our stem, and the Navy's *Benevolence* at our bow. At night great spotlights illuminate their gleaming white sides, the red crosses fanning a common bond among the three different services.

The sickest of the patients are still being carried aboard. There seems to be no end to the P.O.W. liberation, and according to the prisoners themselves, "They haven't begun to touch the camps yet."

The ones who have been here a day or two are beginning to relax. Their eyes are losing that uncomprehending stare. They kid the nurses a little now and then, and have lost their docile obedience. But they watch the Japanese workers from their deck chairs with almost no bitterness. It was as though hatred required energy they cannot waste.

The 11th Airborne—those irrepressible paratroopers who ate us out of house and home the first night we were in Japan—have been determined to produce a brass band to welcome the prisoners of war. We laughed at them about it, but they said, "O.K., you wait. We'll have that band ready within a week."

Tonight, just one week later, they appeared at the processing center in splendid array, musically tooting on a complete set of band instruments. The concert was a great success.

September 8. Little by little, the men are emerging from their cocoons. This morning there was an undercurrent of laughter on the ward for the first time. Interest in food is more than theoretical now. They're able to retain it and cheat like fury to get more than they should. It's for their own good, of course, that we limit them in these first days of hospitalization.

But four years of stealing food to live has made them skillful at it, and they smuggle in "seconds" in spite of our best efforts to prevent it. You find food hidden under pillows, in pajama pockets, everywhere. They lie in bed planning the amazing combinations of food they will eat, back in the States.

So many of the patients have diseases I've known only from textbooks. And almost all have horrible skin infections. "Scabies" and "beri beri" or "pellagra" are an additional diagnosis on almost all of them. Eyesight is seriously affected by the long-standing nutritional deficiencies, and the need for dental work is appalling.

There are blind patients among the prisoners—men who have a total loss of vision from their vitamin deficiencies. They were given no consideration by the Japanese because of their handicap; they had to shift for themselves or die. Where I have known blinded patients who have to be persuaded to feed themselves and be independent, these blind ex-prisoners scramble for chow alertly and are constantly on the ball to see that they receive their share. They learn their way about the wards quickly and rely on no one.

One thing the men simply can't get over is the way supplies are "wasted." For four long years neither they nor their captors wasted a single scrap of paper or shred of tobacco. We passed out chocolate milk in paper cups this morning to save the work of washing glasses. The patients were horrified when the corpsmen collected and threw out the cups.

September 12. This morning I listened to survivors of Bataan and Corregidor tell of their last days before the surrender, of the hopelessness of the struggle, of their desperate hunger, of the wounded and dying who lay outdoors for days because it was impossible to get them to the improvised hospital. And when they finished telling about it, they asked, "How did the people back home take it? Did they figure we let them down? We tried like hell, but we were licked from the minute we started."

It's good to see them growing stronger every day. Men who couldn't walk when they were brought in are sitting on the edge of their beds, talking about the quantities of food they can consume. You can't possibly imagine what meal time looks like among men who have almost starved to death. Secure now in the knowledge that there are unlimited supplies, they still can't overcome the urge to snatch at every passing morsel. The patients are almost relaxed now during the rest of the day, but the appearance of food almost makes animals of them again.

September 16. The admiration of the men on Corregidor and Bataan for General Wainwright is something to see. MacArthur they dismiss contemptuously. "Sure, if they ordered him out, he probably had to go. But they can have him. Give me old Skinny Wainwright, who knows how to stick it out. When we finally surrendered on Bataan and Corregidor, you know what he said? 'I surrendered because I knew there was no way out. But you men never would have, I know. You'd have fought as long as there was one of you alive and I realize it. The surrender was *my* responsibility because I couldn't make men needlessly die any longer!' The other brass would have said, 'I could have held out, but the men let me down.'"

They're beginning to take freedom for granted now, and they feel they're really "up on the news." Now and then they still get a surprise. Last night we borrowed the movie "Here Come the Waves." The word "Waves" held no significance—their six-day educational program had not included mention of a female Navy. They roared with delight during the show; so that was what the Navy had descended to without them? No leaves now, when they returned—get them back on duty, quick! And the Army men, quick to heckle them about the "glamour gobs," were crushed to find that they were the proud possessors of a corps of "Wacs."

September 17. We drove down into the country today at 15 miles an hour in a charcoal-burning autobus. Really a contraption. Out there you realize what the bombing has done. The Japanese look at you and, looking back, you lose all sense of hatred and revenge, and are stirred by nothing but pity. The sight of an old woman poking among the ruins of what was once her home does something to you. They live in gypsy fashion now, but what lies ahead this winter?

There seems no answer to it, for when winter comes the shelter cannot care for all. Even more than the sight of combat casualties, the sight of bombed-out civilians drives home the horror of war. God, how I wish every person on earth had to see it for himself. Even then I suppose war would be done away with for no longer than the generation required to build new armies, new strategies, and new quarrels.

November 11. We left Japan today. Most of the minor headaches of ward management have been smoothed out, and patients are gaining weight and amusing themselves mightily.

November 22. At Manila there were troop ships loading at the same wharf where we took on our additional patients. Our own passengers lined up along the rail to watch the men embark and then returned to their wards almost glowing with satisfaction. "Rugged, this deal," they said loftily as they eased themselves into bed, lounging comfortably, while sipping a glass of chocolate milk. "You got to feel sorry for those guys, not knowing how to come home from the war in style."

Everyone, patients and staff alike, is looking forward to discharge in the near future—and to Christmas at home, and that, of course, contributes to the gala air aboard ship. Morale, which crawled downward as the ship sailed for Manila, made an abrupt change when we pointed toward home, and at the moment is reaching an all-time high.

For the *Marigold*, it's the end of the war, and an epoch is nearly over.

January, 1946. For me and for a number of my colleagues the war was not really over. I sent this "Open Letter from Members of the Army Nurse Corps" to the *American Journal of Nursing:*

"The majority of Army nurses who served overseas during the war years have now accumulated the necessary points for discharge.

"In the midst of a mass movement toward civilian status which resembles the rush for a nylon line, a rather large group of us have elected to remain in the service for the time being. We have been variously laughed at, and been berated by our departing colleagues as 'unwilling to face the future.'

"'Security' is one of the greatest inducements the Army offers its service men and women, yet because we wish this to be a discussion of the professional aspects of Army nursing, we mention this advantage only in passing. It is there, and we who enjoy its benefits are fortunate, yet almost unanimously we disclaim it as a prime motive for staying in.

"Why, then, are we here? The reply is worded in a variety of phrases but the essence is the same. We are here because we sincerely believe that for this year and for the years in the immediate future, the Army Nurse Corps offers nursing opportunities in the field of post-traumatic casualty care unrivaled in any phase of civilian nursing (and we devoutly hope never to be equaled again in the future of our own Army). We are here, because we wish to be a part of the Army Medical Corps program of reconstructive surgery.

"In combat zones, in field and evac and general hospitals in every theater of war, we saw and had a part in the finest lifesaving program the world has ever known. In that program, the essence of its lifesaving power was speed—speed in collecting, speed in transporting, and speed in caring for casualties. That the rapid care of combat casualties paid off with an all-time low mortality rate is now an historic fact. In retrospect, even the mud, and the ever present 'moving again,' and the long hours, and the dozens of little inconveniences fade out into the over-all picture. Someone has said 'an adventure is an inconvenience, rightly considered.'

"Inevitably, the rapidity of patient evacuation in wartime produced one great disadvantage. We cared for thousands but they were 'Patients' not 'individuals.'

"The endless stream has ceased to arrive in daily trainloads, but those who came to us via North Africa and Italy, France and Germany, via Wake and New Guinea, the Philippines and Okinawa, the veterans of every theater of war, are with us still. We know them now, lying patiently month after month in the general hospitals back home. No longer anonymous, blanket-wrapped figures on dirty litters, but individuals—American soldier-survivors of an already-hazy era of combat, who still have to face the aftermath of war.

"Amputations and blindness, paralysis, and plastic reconstruction are with us still. The same people to whom we wanted so much to give that extra moment's time, overseas, are on our wards today. They still have Army time in Army hospitals ahead of them. So have we.

"There is nothing altruistic about the decision. Caring for these soldiers through their various phases of elective surgery and reconditioning will be too worth-while professionally for us to deliberately turn it down.

"We find a deep satisfaction in the knowledge (so often missing in civilian hospitals) that, regardless of wealth or rank, we are able to give the utmost in care to the patients who need it. In the Army, there are no private patients or ward patients—there are only seriously ill patients or patients who are convalescing or are in other stages of progress.

"And last but perhaps most important of all, in the Army the general staff nurse commands respect. Her pay and her rank and her status as an individual are not dependent upon the outside world's insistence that if a nurse be at all capable she must 'better herself' and teach or supervise, or if she must do bedside nursing, she must at least 'special.' The civilian general staff nurse is often not looked up to, or not adequately paid. But we—all of us who like bedside nursing and who delight in the satisfaction of working on a busy ward at the kind of nursing we enjoy, and at the professional level which we believe in—are finding these opportunities daily on Army hospital staffs.

"We gripe, of course, and with cause, at petty annoyances and inconvenient Army rules or traditions; and at many posts we still gaze enviously at the starched white uniforms of our civilian colleagues, muttering about 'the glamour of these seersucker jobs.' But in the final analysis, we're in because we want to be, and we believe we're lucky to be staying."

Percy Jones General Hospital, Battle Creek, Michigan, 1946-47

In the rush to provide sufficient hospital facilities for the continuing stream of casualties returning from both the European and Pacific theatres, the Army commandeered civilian-owned hotels and luxury sanitoria, which were hastily converted into military general hospitals of enormous capacity. Following the war's end and my return to the States I was transferred from the about-to be decommissioned Hospital Ship *Marigold* to the luxury sanatorium in Battle Creek, Michigan, which had previously been a health-food spa for rich dieters and was now a great military Rehabilitation Center. Here I spent my final eighteen months of Army nursing.

February 12, 1946. The Michigan snow and sleet are driving against my window with needle sharpness. But what care I, enjoying the splendor of this new home they call Percy Jones General Hospital. The entire first floor has been left as it was with sun rooms, palm gardens, and fountains, but now with wheelchairs banked six deep.

Almost all the personnel, and of course, all the patients, have returned from overseas. At dinner the thousand or more officers, enlisted men and patients—we all eat together—wear uniforms glowing with brightly-colored theatre ribbons, service patches and military decorations.

I'm working on a 100-bed amputation ward. Most of the patients are leg amputees, but nearly one-third have lost an arm and a few are blind or otherwise additionally handicapped. They are still undergoing extensive surgery, although some have been fitted with prosthesis and are learning to use them. As at Mitchel Field, the wards are cheerful places, although the exuberance of the newly-returned soldier has given way to a sort of jovial cynicism, a reckless "to hell with the world, I have nothing more to lose" attitude. It is born of boredom, spoiling, and an overlong period of hospitalization. But these are the same likeable G.I.s I have known before, a trifle more reserved and harder to know, conforming externally to the accepted G.I. pattern, and all using it to conceal highly individualized thoughts, ambitions, and emotions.

April 11. Several of the men had passes to town last night. I came upon them during the afternoon, seated legless in wheelchairs, with their well-shod prosthetic legs lined up in front of them like soldiers on parade. They were shining their shoes for the evening ahead. There was a louder clamor on this occasion for new socks, an item of equipment for which they had had no use for many months.

You can always put an end to complaints and start an uproar of derision by calling out brightly, "O.K., heroes—would you be interested in buying some Victory Bonds to help the wounded veterans in our Army hospital?" "Buy a bond to help our heroes" is our favorite slogan, followed closely by "Write your Congressman, veteran, the people are behind you."

May 27. I've moved five miles away to the hospital annex at Fort Custer, where the rehabilitation center for patients with spinal cord injuries is maintained.

Cord cases feel a terrible hopelessness: their handicap is far more enduring than the amputees. In earlier years, they would have been doomed to an existence in bed or chair, because they are permanently paralyzed from the site of the injury downward.

Yet their days are crowded with preparation for the future. The goal is for each patient to care for himself completely; hopefully, to learn to walk with crutches, and to be equipped to earn a living, on crutches or from a wheelchair.

They are working to attain a hitherto undreamed-of degree of independence by use of special equipment built into their beds, their tubs, sinks, and toilets. Every ounce of arm muscle-power now provides motion that would formerly have been denied them. There are wheelchair radio repair shops in several locations, equipped with small work units.

An unusual course offered to some of the patients in wheel-chairs is in making flower arrangements. One of the men on my ward comes from a family who has a flower farm in Wisconsin. They have always sold to florists but never before thought of open-ing a retail shop.

The gags and nonsense on the ward are generally good for these patients, but their long-term outlook is not a happy one.

Well, you can always joke about it. "O.K., Goldbrick, roll over."

"Lookit! What am I paying you, nurse, for this service? Raised your salary twice in the last week, didn't I?"

"Kind sir, this Army nurse thanks you for the two extra Cokes provided by your largess."

"If you didn't have me to take care of, you'd be unemployed."

"Oh, noble employer, I'm more than grateful for the endless practice you give me in bed changing. It is becoming a finely developed art."

"Listen, Lieutenant, it's wet again! I'm sorry as hell. God, what a way to spend your life. Cory was right this morning. We should all have been left to die. This way we're no good to anyone."

October 21. The cord patients have been discharged from the Army and transferred to a Veterans' Hospital. Many of them had not been out of their wards for a year or more. I have started to work on a new service—facial reconstructive plastic surgery.

I knew Sim Caldwell on Ward 21 at Mitchel Field a year and a half ago. He was then a pretty sorry-looking soldier. You knew when you took the bandages off his head and surveyed the burned-out mess that was left that whatever happened to him must have been pretty awful. There was not much face under the bandages, no nose, no ears and little mouth, but in the midst of the wreckage two bright eyes looked out at you with interest.

Bad as it was, Sim's facial injury was not his only surgical problem. His right leg had been burned to a crisp and his left one was gone entirely. And his hands were not functional either; they were sensitive, painful claws. That was a long time ago when I knew him on Ward 21.

"They do great work in plastic surgery nowadays," he said confidently. "You won't know me the next time we meet, Lt. Schwartz!" He was right. I didn't. He was transferred to my ward at Percy Jones this week after all these months of hospitalization. I walked on the ward one morning and a familiar voice rang out. "Why, Lt. Schwartz, what are *you* doing here? Gosh, it's good to see you again."

Thirty-five trips to the operating room (yes, thirty-five!) had given Sim the semblance of a face. The badly-burned leg had healed. His hands, no longer claws, are useful again and he manages crutches well with them. The stump of his other leg has provided his toughest setback. It was burned so badly that even now, doctors say it will be another year before a prosthesis can be fitted to it. That's hard to take. "I'll be a permanent fixture in an Army hospital, waiting for that, Lieutenant."

January 6, 1947. It is midnight and I have just come off duty. Tonight, like so many other nights, was a constant and hectic rush with a convoy of patients arriving from a general hospital several states away. It is hard to realize that the war is so long over, that more than a year has passed since V-J Day.

Many of the patients with more than eighteen or twenty months of pain and loneliness behind them are not able to be with their families for even short holidays. Surgeons still carry wartime operating schedules and night nurses are working a seven-day week, just as we did at the height of the combat period.

I wish that everyone in America had to spend the day in such a place as this right now. I think it would be very hard for them to refer thoughtlessly to another war if they could see this one still going on. And it would be a strong object lesson to the grabbers and "me firsters" of the country to watch the patience and quiet determination of wounded men overcoming handicaps of blindness and paralysis and loss of limbs.

I met Artie in the hall on the way to supper. Artie, whom I have admired since Mitchel Field days, is walking well now, on his two new legs, in spite of blindness, and no handicap has ever affected his sunny smile.

We talked for a moment and Artie got out of his wheelchair, standing very tall and straight. "This is the way it ought to be," he said, contentedly. "For ages your voice has been coming down to me as you leaned over the bed to talk. But now I can look down at you when we walk together." Later this evening one of our older men was told that fourteen months of effort to save his leg had been fruitless; bone grafts and plastic work had been in vain.

After lights were out I made my way around the ward giving medications, and as the flashlight's beam revealed row after row of plaster casts, dressings and strange traction devices, I wondered how many thousands of other nurses were still making rounds on wards, all over the world, filled with wartime casualties.

I stopped at a bedside to give a shot of penicillin and the light fell on the book the patient had been reading. It was a biography of Lincoln and the book was open at the Second Inaugural Address. The dim rays fell on the penicillin tray and the syringes, the sleeping soldiers, and the ghostly bandages. And the same rays fell on the final paragraph of the address.

"With malice toward none, with charity for all, with firmness in the right as God gives us to see the right, let us strive to finish the work we are in; to bind up the nation's wounds, to care for him who shall have borne the battle, and for his widow and his orphan—to do all which may achieve a just and lasting peace among ourselves and with all nations."

It seemed an appropriate spot in which to re-read the words. I thought about it for a long minute, then pushed in the penicillin needle firmly, and, tray in hand, finished the rounds.

Chapter 3

Public Health Nursing in Sweden

After leaving Percy Jones and the Army Nurse Corps, I went back to work as a staff nurse in Red Hook, Brooklyn. At night I was completing my interrupted studies in public health nursing at New York University.

One requirement I came up against was "a field experience in an official government agency." Because I was already familiar with the New York City Health Department, I sought this new field work in international health and so became the first American exchange nurse in public health in rural Sweden.

It was scarcely three years after World War II and most of Europe was still recovering. Sweden was prosperous enough to welcome displaced persons and each community had a number of Polish and German Jewish newcomers. Even in Sweden there were still shortages—gas, meat, coffee.

But so good was the cooking, and so ingenious, that an outsider could live entirely unaware of rationed foods. All dairy products, fish and vegetables were plentiful; sugar was scarce but evenly distributed to all in reasonable amounts.

Meat (except pressed meats and processed meat products) was almost unobtainable, though, even with the proper ration points. The people felt this quite acutely. I, in my innocence, hardly noticed it as I consumed divine egg and cheese dishes and vegetables better than any I had ever eaten.

In contrast to the subway and streetcars by which public health nurses got around in New York City, the nurses of rural Sweden, in those post-war, gas-poor days, often traveled by bicycle. That was how I usually made home visits in the suburbs of Rimbo, a rolling farm area about an hour north of Stockholm.

April 12, 1948. I reached the town of Rimbo in lilac time, when the massive white and purple blooms hung thick in every garden. Rimbo is a typical Swedish country village with a population of 2,074 widely spread across the rolling countryside. The paved roads are winding, and the houses—mostly stucco—at first glimpse all seemed to belong to people of a single, comfortable income bracket. Later, I found that this was far from true, but the houses of the poorer families are as attractive and as neatly kept as any others.

This is *"Distriktskoterska Doris"* (*Ameikanse*) now. It's pronounced Schwester Dorice and it seems to me the entire town of Rimbo has phoned or called in the past 24 hours to make sure the visitor had arrived safely.

At the district Health Center I am welcomed by my hostesses and supervisors, *Forsta distriktskoterska Greta*; Miss Johnson, public health nursing supervisor, and *Skoterska* Ingrid, public health midwife. Sister Greta is a live-wire sort of person, cheerful, efficient and full of fun. Sister Ingrid is so startlingly beautiful that she takes your breath away. I have seldom seen a lovelier, healthier-looking woman. She positively radiates friendliness and does this, I notice, with everyone to whom she speaks—the patients, the grocer's boy, the passing townsfolk. Sister Greta speaks very good English, Sister Ingrid none at all. This is an excellent incentive for me to start learning Swedish.

All of us live at the Health Center in a pleasant building, indistinguishable from the private homes surrounding it. Here are to be found the antepartal clinic (which on certain days becomes the child health station), the midwife's and the district nurse's office, and two attractive living units—each a complete apartment by itself. In one of these apartments Sister Ingrid and her husband live; in the other, Sister Greta. Each has a charmingly furnished bedroom, living room, kitchen and bath. In the building next door, I occupy the apartment of the dentist's family, since the town is-for the summer—between dentists, with a new one coming in October.

Upstairs in the Health Center is the Rimbo Maternity Hospital, where all normal deliveries are cared for by the registered public health midwife. Patients who have shown any deviations from the normal are routed to the hospital in Stockholm or a neighboring city. The maternity unit is beautifully equipped and furnished with a nursery (six bassinets), Delivery Room, two three-bed rooms, a sun porch, bath, kitchen and formula room.

Above are quarters for the three nurse's aides and the second public health midwife, whom I have not yet met as she is out of town on leave. The whole center is spotlessly clean, and the obstetrical technique seems to be the equal of that in any full-sized metropolitan hospital. Patients are kept ten days after a first delivery, five or six for their subsequent ones.

April 15. Today I went on rounds with Sister Greta; every aspect of the visit could have been Brooklyn V.N.A. Except for this foolish barrier of language, I might have been out at the Cialinos with Mrs. White, or at 98 Atlantic Avenue with Miss Lebofsky. The work is definitely "official agency": ten schools, tuberculosis control, maternal and child health and venereal disease work. But Greta's actual visits in the home are largely demonstration. Her sleeves are rolled up and she's deep in work. The patients think she's wonderful. You can tell it by their pleasure when she knocks. Everyone knows her, and she hails cyclists on the street, school kids playing ball, housewives in grocery stores.

There are many displaced persons from German prison camps within the district. The mother of the premature twins whom we visited today was one of these. As she offered to shake hands, she displayed a large Nazi prison number indelibly tattooed across her forearm—a grim reminder of the years which make this Swedish freedom seem priceless.

In any event, in the home of another refugee, a charming and intelligent Pole, I was introduced with the usual explanation that I didn't yet speak Swedish. The woman spoke English very well and we fell into excited conversation, I meanwhile admiring her lovely baby. She told me of Sister Greta's kind interest and of the excellent care she'd had from Sister Ingrid. And she wanted to know exactly where I worked.

I said New York and she beamed happily. Taking out a picture of another healthy baby and a letter in Polish, she translated her sister's enthusiastic praise of the visiting nurse who came to help her with her baby. The address was a Manhattan one. Her visits must have been by the Visiting Nurse Service of New York. It made the distance from Sweden to America seem very small and the two concentration camp exiles and their infants, very close.

It is 1 a.m. and I must stop. Although one lamp is lighted in the room, it would be entirely possible to write without it, for this is the season of the midnight sun, and even as far south as Stockholm it is never more than early dusk throughout the night. The wonderful hour just before sunset lasts from 5 p.m. until 11. Then it becomes a little darker and it will now grow steadily brighter till the morning.

April 26. All the experiences of this orientation week in Swedish District Nursing have been delightful. We vary our schedule in much the way it is done at home. At present, Sister Greta is covering two districts, Rimbo and Karsta, and therefore divides her time accordingly. Two days each week are spent at Karsta, one at the clinic there for a child health station session (with the doctor) and one without him for necessary weekly treatments (injections, irrigations and instructions). Both of these clinical periods are in the morning. On the day of the Child Health Clinic, Sister Ingrid also accompanies us to see the pre-natal patients.

In the afternoon, we make home visits throughout the countryside. These could be in any country place at home: a colostomy dressing here, a T.B. visit there, a call to see a mother who has broken several appointments at the Child Health Station. Always the visit is a well-prepared and competently executed one: friendly, easy going and a bit more formal in externals than the ones we make at home. For example, one knocks and says, "Good Morning," and then, as a necessary ceremony, shakes hands with every member of the family. The little boys bow, and the little girls curtsy, and this is done with equal charm in the poorest homes and the finest ones we visit.

Next the visit itself is made. Any Swedish nurse would be at home in Brooklyn and vice versa. (Except that only our most ideal patients at home would be apt to be so completely attentive and cooperative in carrying out the details. Here it is assumed that an occasional mother will fail to respond in such a manner, as indeed they do, but that this will happen only if she is of low intelligence and needs more patient teaching.)

After the visit comes the invariable invitation to coffee, the polite refusal, and the farewell ceremony of handshaking. Even in the clinic, one greets and takes leave of every patient in this manner. The doctor does it also. It is perhaps a bit more time consuming, but it lends great dignity to the visit and one could hardly be rude or inattentive to a patient (or the patient to the clinic personnel) after such a pleasant introduction.

For Kosta and the outlying sections of Rimbo, we use the car. But gasoline is so difficult to obtain that wherever it is feasible, we prefer to hike or cycle. The cycling is wonderful—down long sweeps of sun-lighted country roads, with breathtaking scenery in every direction.

Swedish people love to cycle. In most European countries the cycle is a means of transportation but in Sweden it is recreation also. You have the feeling that many of the routine tasks of life are recreation for the Swedish people. They laugh and sing snatches of folk songs as they whiz by, pedalling furiously.

What I love most of all are these days of "bicycle nursing." One takes a lunch of bread and cheese along, and about midday asks of a Swedish country householder a question, the translation of which is, "Will you do me the honor to permit my lunching in your yard, please?"

And then one stretches out luxuriously beneath a pine tree in the warm, fragrant sunshine to devour a sandwich and a cookie. And often the housewife fixes sandwiches quickly for her own family and they join you on a picnic. And on such occasions the answer to the routine question, "Will you stay for coffee?" is no longer negative and the good coffee is shared between the picnicking nurses and the picnicking household.

Such a generous spirit is doubly significant, for *coffee*—that most treasured of all the Swedish foods—is, after all, still rationed. it is no longer served at meals, but is taken once daily, in the afternoon or evening with due ceremony, often out of doors. And to be invited to share the daily coffee ration, as we often are, is kindness itself.

May 10. At the Professional Women's Club in nearby Nortalja tonight, I sat between fluent interpreters, Sister Greta and the high school German teacher, who spoke a very comprehensive English learned in Germany. Here in the rural area, because both nurses and teachers are relatively few in number, they meet jointly for professional matters, community activities and recreation.

It might have been any good Women's Club at home. They conduct meetings according to Robert's Rules of Order. The members speak with poise and interest and the group is addressed by an outside speaker on a book of current interest. Afterward there is such a supper as would bowl over any cook I know, and then, with the love of gaiety which seems to characterize every party here, a gathering around the piano for the lusty singing of folk songs. This evening, they even hauled out a book called *American Community Songs,* and with the solemn attitude one associates with the rendering of a foreign national anthem, they proceeded through all nine verses of "My Darling Clementine." Then the good ladies ended their gala evening by mounting their iron steeds in very dressed-up clothing and rolled down the hillside as they called, "Adjio, Adjio."

June 1. Tomorrow I go to Stockholm to the International Congress of Nurses meetings. The papers here are full of the event, for it is the largest international meeting ever to have been held in Sweden. Four thousand nurses are expected from every comer of the world. I shall be in Stockholm for one week and then return to Rimbo, for another six weeks' apprenticeship.

In Sweden, nurses really have achieved professional status. They do not use the word as much as we do in America but because of their participation in national as well as community life, the people of their country look upon them with respect as civic leaders. And so, when they announced themselves hostesses to an international gathering of their colleagues, every city in Sweden extended an invitation to the nurses of the foreign nations to be their guests and wander where they pleased, inspecting not only medical facilities but every aspect of Swedish life—schools, homes, industries, universities, historical institutions and housing projects. "For in this way," said the lay people of the country, "you will see how the work of the nurse and the life of the community overlap, and you will understand the reasons why we think of our nurses as highly as we do."

The National Railroads offered transportation free of charge, as a tribute to the Swedish nurses; the Swedish Medical Association made a gift of money to enable the National Nurses Association to pay the way of delegates from the war-devastated European countries who otherwise could not have come. And since Stockholm is a relatively tiny city for such a gathering, Swedish doctors, lawyers, and political leaders as well as hundreds of ordinary citizens put their own homes at the disposal of the nurses' organization to house 4,000 guests. As for the feeding of such a multitude, the women of Stockholm—volunteers, mind you—have set up a restaurant in an enormous auditorium and cook and serve 8,000 meals a day (and wash the dishes afterward, just in time to begin doing it all over again).

Taxi-drivers, street car conductors, people who meet you on the street, smile and say, "Welcome to Stockholm. May it be a profitable meeting."

June 6. A group of nurses went to the Royal Palace with Miss Gerda Hojer, President of the International Council of Nurses and a member of Parliament. In an entirely unscheduled appearance, the ninety-two-year-old King came out, and shaking hands with Miss Hojer, displayed a knowledge of nursing problems that would have done credit to a university teacher in a nursing department. Furthermore, he was entirely familiar with the agenda of the meetings, as were most of the Swedish people.

June 7. Frau Blunck, close to seventy now, is engaged in the task of re-organizing the German Nurses Association (disbanded by Nazi order in 1940).

My own feelings during our hour-long talk were very mixed; it is impossible not to admire the job which she is doing. I find it just as impossible to share her firm conviction that Germany was a martyr country which the world used as a buffer to fend off the threat of Soviet Russia.

We switched from politics to health care trends. Here Frau Blunck was well informed. We discussed modern trends in rehabilitation, plastic surgery, what each of our country's veteran's hospitals has done with paraplegics. Again I felt a queer, sinking feeling in the pit of my stomach—the same feeling which I had when we used German prisoners of war for hospital corpsmen, during the war years.

Here we sat today, each rejoicing in the triumph of rehabilitation which our hospitals are achieving, yet a short five years ago, each of us was backing with every ounce of energy, opposing philosophies which were causing this destruction. And each of us took comfort in the thought that we were nurses engaged in "creative" and not "destructive" work.

I thought of the days at the close of the war, when the ambulance planes rolled in with ghosts of men released from concentration camps. We turned to other topics. Frau Blunck spoke of the Valley of the Rhine in springtime. "It must be beautiful," I said. "My brother has told me it was the greenest country he had ever seen."

Frau Blunck was enthusiastic instantly. "Your brother—he has been to Germany? He knows my country?"

"Yes," I said and changed the subject. How could I say, "His infantry division spearheaded the crossing of the Rhine. Perhaps they helped to bomb your home to the shreds you tell me of." And again I had that terrible sinking feeling. How does one feel toward an elderly German colleague who says, "There was nothing else to do but go along with Hitler. It was survival."

How does one feel toward a colleague who gave every ounce of her strength to the work of elevating nursing standards (a commendable trait if ever there was one), a nurse who looks at you and speaks with a sincerity that is unmistakable.

"Sister Doris, it is not possible for you to understand what this month in Sweden means to me. It is not possible to understand and I pray that you may never know. In ten years, this is the first time I have not been hungry. There is not a single night when most of the people in Germany are not hungry, even today."

June 15. I am back at the rural town of Rimbo. Now for a quick run-through of Swedish Rural District Nursing.

In Sweden, where 90 percent of the nurses are employed by county governments, it is customary for attractive housing to accompany a public health nurse's job. When a nurse or a midwife marries, the couple frequently continues to occupy the wife's apartment. I once attended a social gathering in a nearby town at which the husbands of the nurses present badgered the husband of the hostess for a hint just before his wife retired. "For," said one craftily, "everyone knows that yours is by far the most spacious and best-planned apartment in the Landet (county), and with just a small bit of advance information, I am quite sure I could persuade my wife to ask for a transfer to this district." The wives pooh-poohed this; transfers and districts were professional matters in which they brooked no interference from their spouses.

The more time I spend with Sister Greta, the more I am convinced that she could swap jobs with anyone on the staff at home.

June 22. I have been much interested in our Maternity Center here. The midwives deliver even the private patients who have had a doctor for pre-natal care. Their technique is excellent (three years of nursing plus two years at the State College of Midwifery), and there is not much fuss about the having of the baby.

The mother arrives, in labor, is greeted by her friend, the midwife, whom she has seen regularly throughout her pregnancy, and is welcomed by the other patients, who are neighbors and old friends. The mothers are far more relaxed than mothers in a hospital at home.

Although Grantly Dick Read's philosophy has not reached Rimbo in quotation marks, his teachings are instinctively carried out. When the mother has had her baby, there is such general rejoicing at the center that one would think she was the first of her species to have accomplished such a feat. Papa arrives, is beamed at, congratulated and given coffee. Everybody is happy over every single birth, like members of a family.

The good in such a system makes you almost forget that blood is not stocked at this center, that no obstetrician is available locally in case an emergency occurs, and that although the fine hospitals of Stockholm are not too far away, they might be too far sometime, though that has never happened in the history of the center. At worst, persistent bleeders have been taken to the city by ambulance, and so far, they have always responded successfully to treatment.

But then there are still many areas in the United States where blood and skillful obstetricians are not available. And they don't all have the splendid little health centers of Swedish rural communities or the well-trained nurse-midwives either.

July 1. I suddenly found myself engaged in the self-same activity which July lst had found me in for years, i.e., chaperoning a busload of exuberant youngsters en route to a summer holiday. The fact that they spoke another language hardly mattered; the same group of mothers was gathered at the station, the one inevitably home-sick child who didn't want to go wailed mournfully on the platform, and as always, a greenish-looking cherub got carsick on the bus. In certain particulars, all countries are alike and getting children off to summer camp is surely one of them.

And what a lovely camp they had! This camp I visited took thirty-five children ages five to ten (both boys and girls) and was beautifully planned and built for tiny children.

The summer camp program was begun here many years ago for underprivileged city children. With the extension of Sweden's social welfare program, it has gradually been expanded until free summer holidays are now available for all but the very top income youngsters. A small portion of the funds is derived from local sources, but by far the greater portion comes from the tax on matches.

Since the tax has been imposed, matchboxes bear the picture of a happy youngster playing in the sunshine and the word *Solsticken*, which means literally "stick of sunshine." Thus the "Sunshine Camps" came into being, and these are supported by the Swedish people.

The state discourages large camps for this vacation holiday; it is the consensus of opinion that small groups under careful supervision will get more benefit. This automatically eliminates the more elaborate and stimulating programs of many American summer camps, and gives the Swedish variety more of a congenial "family relationship" aspect.

I kept thinking of the camp registration in New York last May, of the mothers who waited at the social agencies only to be turned away, of Miss Berry (my supervisor) wheedling arrangements for especially needy youngsters from her social worker friends, of how even with everyone working cooperatively, only a fraction of the children could be taken.

July 9. The home I saw for the infirm aged in Norrtalje was wonderful. Imagine, if you can, a cheerful, homey place, built like a boarding house or family dwelling unit, where every sunny room is easily available for nursing care, but totally lacking a hospital atmosphere.

Trailing vines and blooming plants covered the walls. The beds all had hand rails and overhead trapezes to help their occupants in and out. Bedside tables adjusted easily to "tray" and "reading" positions and in addition, like most Swedish bedside tables, contained a locked compartment for the patient's personal papers and things she didn't want handled by the nurse. These also had a long drawer for knitting materials and a safe for eyeglasses and false teeth, beside the usual full-size table drawer. Each bed had an adjustable reading lamp and call light.

The dining room and living room were planned for wheelchair guests. Ramps with tracks for beds or wheelchairs led to a lovely garden (all Swedish hospitals have readily accessible gardens for their patients and most of them have a private park arrangement for the nurses). Norrtalje's T.B. clinic is in a fortunate position— probably one which is equalled by few T.B. clinics elsewhere, even in Sweden. For it was the center for one of the Government's mass X-ray surveys recently, and so cooperative was the population, so thorough the propaganda and so efficient the public health nurses' follow up that to the best of their knowledge, every case of T.B. in the entire area is known and under treatment at the present time, every suspicious prospect is under constant watching and every arrested case is coming in for regular supervision.

Thus it is for the moment at least—a wholly prophylactic teaching clinic. It continues on a busy schedule: X-raying contacts, new arrivals in the community, persons released from supervisory care in institutions. But in this district at the present time T.B. is well-controlled.

I am interested in the provision for the nurses' summer holidays (one month). Since there is an acute shortage of public health nurses, the holiday means that unless a substitute is found, the local health center services must shut down. This is a real disaster to the community, so that many emergency measures are employed. Nurses without State College of Public Health training are occasionally employed for this short time. More often, retired P.H. nurses return to work in their former districts, thoroughly enjoying the month of work.

All Swedish nurses retire on pension at the age of fifty-five but are eligible for a one year at a time extension until the age of sixty. Then no more. After that they are considered ready to plough back into the community in voluntary services the skills and knowledge they have obtained during their years of nursing service.

In any event, as an emergency measure, selected nurses over sixty may now return to pinch-hit during the summer holidays, and this is proving to be an all-around good solution.

July 27. So much happens so quickly that I never seem to get it all on paper. Rural district nursing is no longer a rapid succession of new experiences, but now, after five and a half weeks of it, a fairly stable routine of clinics and home visits, all of which add up to a generally high standard of public health nursing anywhere.

I spent yesterday at the Swedish Nurses' Association getting my August plans mapped out. I leave for Lappland, far beyond the Arctic Circle, to participate in the work at the most northerly Health Station, among the Lapplanders. And then (and this has me so excited that I couldn't sleep last night), a Dutch and a Belgian nurse and I are to accompany the doctor and the Swedish district nurse on a three-day trek (by foot and boat) to the most northerly nomadic Lapps, for whom a clinic will be held.

The fact that I brought no camping clothes and do not own a sleeping bag and rucksack bothered my Swedish plan-makers not at all. "Just borrow them," said they blandly, and so it looks at the moment as though I shall be hiking in Johan's trousers, Greta's lumberjacket, and woollies belonging to the Syster in Norratalje. And sleeping in somebody's uncle's sleeping bag because it's the lightest weight one available.

We leave from Abisko, where the Health Station is. This is the point at which the railroad ends. Tourists in quest of the midnight sun may come this far, but beyond it one may travel only by ski or reindeer sled in winter or on foot during the brief summer thaw.

August 1. This morning we met at the Central Station in Stockholm to start for Lappland to study the work of the Swedish district nurse, Syrana Porcma-Varyura, who promised to take us into the Arctic world and to show us the Lappland health services. The "Dutch and Belgian Nurses" turned out both to be from Holland and to have had Commonwealth Fund Scholarships to the University of Chicago, where they majored in Child Guidance. After this they will return to set up the nursing and social work program in the new child guidance clinics at Amsterdam and the Hague.

They were wonderful women. The Swedish Distriktsyster was beyond description; there are legends about her all over Sweden. The legends are of a tiny (under 5 foot) woodland gnome who is apt to appear any place in the snowy mountains of the north when trouble brews, and who can out-walk, out-climb, and outdo in woodsmanship, the stoutest-hearted Lapp. For over seventeen years Sister Syrena (who was once an operating room supervisor and later an X-ray nurse and therefore must now be almost fifty) has lived alone in Keruna, the most isolated and difficult district in all of Sweden. It is 540 square miles of rocky mountains without a single road included in the area.

Much of this space is uninhabited, of course, but some 3,000 people live in it and among them are several hundred nomad Lapps who are constantly on the move, so that locating them is always difficult. A sort of grapevine keeps them in communication with the outpost telephones possessed by the more home-loving and settled of Syster Syrena's clients, and emergency calls come through in record time.

Answering those calls, however, is a different matter. Syrena goes on foot, racing over snow and river beds and crossing the many lakes in home-made Lapp boats. On such journeys she lives in the sod huts of the natives and they feed her and provide whatever help she needs.

Often a trip takes a week or more, and in the spring, when melting snow and flooded rivers make any kind of travel (including helicopter landing) absolutely impossible, Syrena leaves her home and moves into a Lapp tent or sod hut for six weeks, to be accessible in case of emergency.

During this period the district doctor, who remains in Keruna (south of the melting ice), takes over the work of district nurses in the area which he can reach, and Syrena takes over his work north of the ice jam. They communicate by telephone, but they are absolutely isolated otherwise.

Syrena and the doctor (who loves this area and the job as much as she does) have trained many of the Lapps and Finns in the equivalent of Red Cross First Aid. Locked drug and supply cabinets have been distributed through the area and the keys given to the most trustworthy citizens. Should emergencies occur when neither the nurse nor doctor can make it through the mountains, they direct the care of the patient and his treatment by telephone, using cabinet supplies.

Once a year, in summer, the nurse and doctor make their formal rounds, immunizing babies, checking on chronic patients who "ought to be brought out before the winter," and, most importantly, checking on which citizens will be valuable as "helpers" in the many emergencies to come throughout the approaching winter. It was on a part of this yearly journey that we were to accompany them.

August 6. We took off at 2 a.m. (just as the sun rose over the snow-topped mountains), for this was to be a busy day with many visits. The midwife's husband's pants gave me a slightly square appearance. By the time it should have grown light enough to take our treasured photographs, it had begun to pour, and it rained with the consistency of Noah's Biblical experience for the next four days. Our boots were soaked. We ourselves were soaked, and the Arctic Mountains were turned to knee-deep mud. It didn't faze Syrena and the doctor; apparently they had never taken a trip under different conditions. We plodded on to family after family, now on foot, now by boat, now to a family (usually Finnish) living in isolated splendor in a conventional farmhouse, now to a crowded Lappish family in a tent of reindeer hide or an earthen hut.

The Lapps are a quiet, dignified Scandinavian race, with merry eyes and an air of great inner contentment. Their life is very primitive, but it is so by choice. They are literate people (probably related to the Russians and the Finns, though social anthropologists are not agreed on this) and their way of life is a product of a peculiar brand of Christianity which, like that of the Amish farmers of Pennsylvania, tends to turn them away from the "evils of the modern machine-age world."

They have little crime, little immorality, little T.B. or V.D., and relatively few emotional maladjustments. By law their children must attend Lappish schools where the Swedish school curriculum is in effect, and this means sending the children to Keruna from the first grade upwards to a sort of boarding school.

One of my most unforgettable memories will always be the Lappish hut wherein we ate one noon-time, a grass and dirt affair, with a floor of birch leaves. Stretched out in utter contentment were the doctor, the district nurse and visitors, the baby in a cradle of thong-laced reindeer hide, the small Lapp boys in their brilliant costumes and fantastic scarlet-tasselled hats, and Mama and Papa and a four-teen-year-old girl, equally colorfully arrayed.

Johana, one of the Dutch nurses, said, "I feel as though we're in a play. I keep waiting to hear the audience applaud the scenery."

The friendly but fierce-looking dogs nestled damply against us. Then as I looked up at the rounded earthen walls and ceiling I saw the strange incongruity—the only note of modern "civilization."

On the wall, just where it rounded into the mossy ceiling, there was a twig of birch. And on it, carefully framed in a modernistic dime-store silvered frame, was the graduation picture of the daughter of the family, in which picture some thirty-five Lappish boys and girls were carefully attired in blue suits and fine white "city dresses" for the occasion.

Lapp women almost uniformly go to Keruna for their deliveries at the hospital (and with an eye to the difficulties of transportation in the spring, manage quite successfully to space their pregnancies so that they will not be due during this hazardous period). Those who expect to deliver then must, of course, come to Keruna as boarders before the ice breaks up.

Even this is preferable to delivering in the Arctic winter, and for some years they have had almost 100% of the babies delivered at the hospital. The maternity mortality rate is as low here as in the biggest cities—ditto the infant mortality rate except for premature babies, but even the rate for these is exceptionally low.

The Lapp diet is inadequate, of course, and vitamins and minerals are furnished for the children. However, it has been difficult to educate the parents in the need to use these. Together with insufficient sunlight (it is dark 24 hours a day for six months of the year), the environment and diet are responsible for both scurvy and rickets among pre-school children.

Another ailment peculiar to the Lapps is an intestinal parasite harbored by Lapp dogs and reindeer. The Lapps sleep with their dogs on the birch or pine floors of the cozy huts. They do this for warmth as much as companionship. And the eggs of the parasites, harbored on the hair of the dogs, sometimes are inhaled by humans, producing a lung infection not known to any other people and very difficult to treat. Other than this they are wonderfully healthy. In spite of the simplicity of the life, many of the Lapps are relatively wealthy, for a herd of reindeer has great value and costs them almost nothing but hard work to keep in good condition.

All in all, we visited about seventeen Lapp camps on our trip and since the doctor and Syster Syrena were known to every family, we were welcomed as honored guests.

August 21. The Swedish homemaker, frequently called the home sister, is not a professional person. Her training is carefully planned and supervised, but it is essentially a training in domestic skills. How then does one account for the fact that she is looked up to as a community worker in the field of public health, and that she is beloved by the district nurse and midwife and by the mothers and the children into whose lives she comes in time of need?

Today I talked with Froken Margareta Nordstrom, the human dynamo responsible for the education of these homemakers. Froken Nordstrom is a member of Sweden's Royal Social Board, the supervising authority responsible for the apportionment of state funds which subsidize the service.

The homemaker is found in every section of the country, "to replace the mother in the home in time of childbirth, sickness, or other emergency situation." She is, almost invariably, one of the most popular visitors to the home, for she makes her entrance when a real emergency is present. Her preparation enables her to take over the household tasks with skill and frequently to teach a family what order and system mean in running a home efficiently and pleasantly.

When necessary, the home sister takes over all of the household duties. She is well-compensated for her efforts. Each community provides an attractively furnished apartment for the home sister.

Specifically, the rules provide that she shall be given "one room and kitchen" without cost. She is to be provided with heat, light, and telephone, twenty days of holiday annually, and excellent sickness and pension coverage. She is entitled to free meals at her place of work. In addition, she receives a salary of 2800 kronor a year (about $900) plus bonuses for length of service. Homemakers working in remote northern areas receive an additional sum called a "wilderness bonus."

Competition among communities for the services of a good homemaker has led to the selection of some of the most attractive apartments in the neighborhood for the home sister's use. Several which I visited were as attractive as any occupied by the community's nurses and midwives.

August 24. This morning I arrived in Stockholm at 6 a.m. to begin a dizzying week of sightseeing. By 7 o'clock I was ensconced on a great sailing ship in Stockholm's harbor, which is used as a Youth Hostel, permanently anchored there.

My cabinmates were a vivacious French youngster who is hiking through the Scandinavian countries on her summer holiday, a high school teacher from Finland, here for an educational conference, and a Japanese sociology student, here to do research work in the Swedish Royal Library. We talked at full speed for an hour, had breakfast together and went our various ways. Mine was in the direction of the Swedish College of Public Health, where I was to put in an appearance by 8:30.

At the college I had a chance to clarify my impressions of the "B.C.G." program of vaccination against tuberculosis and to hear its value measured in round figures by some of Sweden's leading doctors. Their reports exceeded even the glowing ones I had expected.

Within the next couple of years, they believe that the entire tuberculin negative part of the population will have been vaccinated, and that this procedure, plus the constant work with Sweden's already infected cases, and the continuation of T.B. detection programs now in force, will make the problem of T.B. a minor one here.

So convinced are they of the efficiency of "B.C.G." on the basis of their own statistics that they no longer leave control groups unvaccinated, since this would be a deliberate and unjustifiable exposure to a condition which they feel could be controlled. The "B.C.G." is voluntary, however, and is still refused because of religious objections by the very small sect of Seventh Day Adventists, which, for the moment at least, affords a sort of control group.

August 26. Last evening, since we were at liberty in Stockholm, we went to hear Sweden's best-loved singers, Jussi and Anna Lisa Bjorling, who sang out of doors in a green and leafy amphitheater. It was wholly lovely. Thousands of people were sitting or lying on the grass, intent on the magnificent program. Across the lagoon, Skansen, the open-air museum, caught the sunset on its rocky cliffs and its great brick tower seemed to be on fire.

Family groups were everywhere; people attend such concerts with their baby carriages or with youngsters sitting placidly in the little rumble-seats with which all Swedish parents' bicycles are equipped. Out in the lagoon a Viking ship propelled by twenty sets of oars (a concession to tourists, but fun, anyway) rolled in the backwash of a speed boat (also a concession to tourists and considerably less desirable aesthetically).

At one point a flight of gulls flew across the sky, their white feathers turned pink and purple in the dying sunlight. Overhead the clouds were puffs of brilliant color, forming a perfect backdrop for the lovely woman who sang. Anna Lisa looks like all the princesses of fairy tales, and sings, together with her husband, with such obvious enjoyment, that it's hard to tell whether they or the audience are the most enthusiastic. After it was over, we took a boat trip around Stockholm's harbor and came back with a full moon following us all the way.

August 28. This morning I went through the thirty miles of corridors of Sodersjukhusset (Sweden's largest general hospital) a second time. The hospital's magnificent facilities are available to everyone alike (Royal family to humblest citizen) at 4 Kronor daily (a little more than $1.00). There are only two-bed and four-bed rooms available for general use, with the decision of which room will harbor whom based entirely on the gravity of the illness. The fee covers every hospital cost, including the doctor.

Since hospital fees are thus largely born by tax funds, you can well understand why the Voluntary Health Insurance rate (covering the small portion of the hospital cost for which the patient is responsible) is so low that any Swedish worker should be able to afford it. A tremendous campaign for 100 per cent membership in the voluntary plan is under way, and it has increased its membership from 20 per cent of Sweden's population to 58 per cent in very little time. There is every expectation of extending it to cover all, long before the date for socialization comes.

To move from the impact of medical care (and the planning for it) as it touches the entire nation to the impact of medical facilities on the individual patient, one needs to see the growing plants and vines—literally thousands of them—that line the walls of every room and corridor. This hospital feels, as do most here, that a profusion of growing plants makes for an atmosphere which is well worth the trouble of caring for them.

With such a setting, cut flowers, which are more time-consuming (and which always arrive at awkward times), can be eliminated on the patients bedside tables, thus making the overall work of "greenhousing" less of a problem, and providing an atmosphere which everyone, patients and personnel, finds enjoyable. Their out-patient waiting room is a joy to enter: comfortable chairs, magazines, and plants galore.

I suspect that what they say is right, "The wear and tear on the rather superior equipment is much less costly in the end, than the wear and tear on personnel caused by unhappy and uncooperative patients."

September 28. It's hard to believe that in only two more days I shall be returning home to Red Hook, there to await Sister Greta's visit, next year, to work in my district, under auspices of the Visiting Nurse Association of Brooklyn. The more time I spend with the Swedish nurses, the more I become convinced that we could easily swap jobs between staff nurses here and staff nurses at home, with profit to both.

Chapter 4

The Frontier Nursing Service

While attending New York University, I elected a second clinical field experience in rural Kentucky, with the Frontier Nursing Service (F.N.S.), the famous "nurses on horseback" who brought safe midwifery and public health nursing programs to an isolated population in Appalachia.

This was still storybook America. I remember the stories galore (and pictures in every nurse's album) of the "stretchering" of patients into town. In such emergencies the neighborliness of mountain people showed at its best.

A message would come into an outpost center, "Hiram's burned and like to die," or "Becky's wasted turrible." The nurse reached the cabin in record time to find a patient who needed medical care, and badly. Her routine orders covered the treatment of emergency situations, but more than that was required. While she prepared her patient for a long and difficult trip, the husband or a youngster went for help to neighboring homes. A home-made stretcher was prepared with poles and blankets.

All the men available were called, for stretchering a heavy patient through the mountains on a slippery and bitter winter night was vastly difficult. Yet it was done repeatedly. At times the litter bearers had to be relieved every four or five minutes all the way, yet there was never a lack of volunteer assistants or personnel to man a raft, or boat, or any other means of transportation when the nurse said, "We'll have to get him to the hospital in Hyden, fast!"

One woman, on her own, began the Service. Mrs. Mary Breckenridge was from a wealthy Southern family which had contributed a vice president and several senators to the United States. She was divorced and a mother of two children who had died in infancy. This was back in the 1920s and wealthy women simply didn't work. But she did not want to live on family money.

Mrs. Breckenridge became a nurse. She rode horseback through the region, finding that the biggest losses among patients were mothers and babies at childbirth. Her work was cut out for her.

The only schools of midwifery were in England at the time, so she studied in the Outer Hebrides and brought back with her British nurse-midwives. She used her influence as a woman of wealth and service to develop committees of leading citizens and debutantes in every U.S. city to raise money for the Service. She offered field experiences to Bennington and Wheaton and other colleges, from which good horsewomen could come to teach the nurses to ride and to care for horses. It became a great adventure. The association of former F.N.S. couriers is worldwide.

The F.N.S. still exists, and college students, men and women, may volunteer for a month of running errands and doing odd jobs. The only horseback riding now, though, is recreational.

December 4, 1949. Got here after a five and a half hour bus trip into the mountains. There is still no railroad in Leslie County and while the war brought a modern highway up from Lexington (to encourage the export of lumber and coal from heretofore inaccessible areas), getting into the mountains is still no easy task. The highway is already in bad repair. One circles and swings around wicked-looking turns, with coal trucks plunging headlong in both directions with no heed to sides of the road or any normal traffic considerations.

There are two directions in which to travel: up and down; scarcely a foot of land is level anywhere. The soil erosion is extreme. Whole mountainsides look ready to tumble down; deep gashes of mud show along the tracks where lumbering has been "successful"; not a blade of grass or twig remains where a forest formerly stood.

Where lumbering and coal extraction have not left their scars, the creeks and rivers have. The bus driver said, "Ain't really whatcha call a flood right now but them creeks is surely UP." I asked him why the people built so near the water.

"All of them houses you see are brand new. Flash floods took 'em all away two years ago. Most people went right back and built exactly where they'd been."

We reached the mining town of Hyden, county seat, and the only town in Leslie County. "Got street lights just last week," the driver said with something like pride. I was the only occupant of the bus.

The main street was two blocks long, cut through by another of equal length. These four blocks were the town. It was copied — exactly—from a Western movie. The dirty helmeted miners in their dungarees were turning into the noisy cafe doorway, their mules standing patiently outside.

The dilapidated, square, rusty-looking courthouse had a tower where a clock once stood, but it had long since fallen off. The mine shafts opened right onto the street, and the dim lights on the miners' hats cut through the dusk. Kentucky at last!

The drugstore-jukebox-general merchandising establishment was also the bus station. There was no one there to meet the bus, so in accordance with instructions, I went inside and asked the clerk to call the Frontier Nursing Service Hospital. "Jeep'll be right down," she said. And, with a great rattling of hood and superstructure, it was.

"Here, you men," yelled the driver, a hefty-looking older woman, to the crowd of miners. "Who's going to give us a hand with this valise?" This was Eva Gilbert, Director of the School of Nurse Midwifery. She was all bustle and energy.

In minutes the Jeep crashed to a halt near the hospital, halfway up a mountain overlooking Hyden. Instantly dogs appeared from every direction, jumping up for a muddy welcome. Everybody has a dog here. Mongrel and thoroughbred, it makes no difference, just so it has four feet and loves you.

Eva and I dislodged the heavy suitcase and stumbled with it through the mud to midwives' quarters near the hospital. "Midwives" is a cheerful sort of dormitory home for students. There are six in the school this term, about all they can take in order to give each the opportunity for a maximum number of deliveries during the six-month training period. All are registered nurses; some hope to work in F.N.S., some come from the foreign mission field.

December 8. Facts, assorted, gleaned in the first few days' conversation with Mrs. B and others: F.N.S. covers approximately 700 square miles of rugged mountain country. Prior to 1941 it was almost impossible to travel in or out except on horseback. Jeeps can now cover the connecting roads between outpost nursing centers in favorable weather; if the creeks and rivers are high, horses are still required. There is not one of the twelve nursing districts where Jeep travel is feasible for reaching a majority of the patients' homes. F.N.S. serves approximately 10,000 people in Leslie County and part of Clay-Owlsley, Perry and at one time a bit of Beverly.

Since 1925 the Frontier Nurses have delivered almost 8,000 mothers in their mountain cabin homes. An 18-bed cottage hospital has been available at Hyden, where abnormal cases, observed throughout the pre-natal period, could be brought up for delivery under the supervision of the Service's resident medical director. Of all those delivered at home or in the hospital, there have been only ten maternal deaths.

At the start of the service this area was without a single physician or registered nurse. There was no motor road in the entire county. Few mountain families had any contact with the outside world, and midwifery was entirely in the hands of untrained "Granny" midwives.

Old statistics on the maternal mortality and infant mortality problems are not available, since registration of births and deaths was not required. In a survey trip prior to setting up F.N.S., Mrs. Breckenridge personally interviewed fifty-three rural midwives, visiting them in their homes and talking to the families where they had carried on their work. None gave postpartum care of any type. Having completed the delivery, they left the home; their job was finished. Prenatal care was quite unknown. None had had any preparation for midwifery except an apprenticeship by helping older midwives. Only four had ever seen a medical book of any kind.

Five untrained and unlicensed mountaineers were discovered using the title of doctor and practicing as physicians. These were frequently called by a midwife who got into trouble with a delivery. Twelve of fifty-three midwives claimed to use silver nitrate in infants' eyes at birth. None of the others had ever heard of this procedure.

The majority "never had to call a doctor yet," and "never lost a mother or a child." Interviews with the families given care produced a very different story. Many midwives reported eclampsia cases happening to other midwives, never to themselves.

All reported postpartum hemorrhage, but only five knew how to hold the fundus. One used a verse from the Bible (Ezekiel 16:6— *"And when I passed by thee, and saw thee polluted in thine own blood, I said unto thee when thou was in thy blood, Live; yea, I said unto thee, when thou was in thy blood, Live"*) to control bleeding and reported that repetition of this also would successfully control hemorrhage in a dehorned steer.

All fifty-three midwives cut the cord with unboiled scissors, greased the area with lard or castor oil, and some used a "clean scorched rag" to dress it with.

December 10. The Wendover nurses, however varied their interests and abilities, have some of the characteristics of a large and well-adjusted family. They are able to enjoy moments of utter nonsense in which simple things seem very funny and are able to switch with ease to focusing attention on books, or music, or politics. There is little about the table-talk to indicate that most of the people gathered here go "out" not more than once a year.

There is a vast amount of good-will and cooperation. Suppose that it is a necessity because of the isolation. One assumes responsibility not only for a job—which, of course, is natural—but for those things which make for easy and pleasant communal living. Some typical additional duties follow:

The feeding and watering of animals at odd times throughout the day, the pinch-hitting at someone else's work from time to time, the assistance with stubborn and untimely household problems "because the cook is sick" or 'because the river rose while one of the girls was home and she couldn't get back on schedule."

December 12. At breakfast, Mrs. B. says to an F.N.S. volunteer from Bennington, "Marcy, Doris must learn to ride." Like that!

Marcy pales a bit and says politely, "Yes, Mrs. Breckenridge."

Mrs. B. says, "By Friday, Marcy. I want her ready to ride District with Anna May by Friday."

Assorted ears prick up around the table. Marcy says politely, "Yes, Mrs. Breckenridge."

I swallow—hard.

As we leave the table Mrs. B. says, "Marcy, when you take Doris out this morning, give it to her!"

By arrangement I meet Marcy at the stable. I see a dim blur of human and a dimmer blur of horse. He smiles—nay, leers at me.

I learn to put on a bridle and a saddle. Tommy's ears lie flat. He's thinking "City Slicker."

I mount. Not gracefully. Dismount. Get on again. Marcy gets her horse. "Come on, let's go," she says.

"You mean— GO?"

We start off down the hill. It's like sitting on top of the Empire State Building in a windstorm. Marcy calls instructions. "Lean back; relax; hold your reins away from the saddle."

We reach the river. "Where do we go to now?" I ask.

Marcy looked surprised. "Across. There isn't any other way to go. "

We enter the river. Tommy pulls like fury. "He's going to roll," I bellow.

"No, he's going to take a drink of water," says Marcy, reasonably. "Let him have his head."

I give him his head and instead of bolting or rolling, he takes a drink of water.

"Maybe they *are* predictable," I reason. At which point Tommy goes round in circles in the river.

"Pull him up," says Marcy. I pull him up. "Now start him straight ahead across the water."

I start him straight ahead. He goes around in a circle. "Tommy," I say firmly, "behave yourself." It comes out: "T-T-Tommy, b-b-be-ha-have your-s-s-s-self." When Tommy tires of walking in circles, he conveys me to the other side. At his own discretion.

"A good first ride develops confidence," says Mrs. B. when we get back. "Don't hold your reins so tightly."

"Dismount," says she.

The space between Tommy and the ground is roughly equal to that covered by a department store escalator.

"Yes, Ma'am," I say. Only suicide could result from such an act, and for the longest time I remain immobile. Getting off at last, I plant my boot firmly on Tommy's rear and thus encourage him to go. At this point, confidence is not exactly a characteristic of either of us.

December 14. My first "real" day was on foot and we followed some of the darndest muddy trails I'd ever seen, wading through creekbeds, sliding down bits of mountain and generally pushing at the project with prodigious energy until we finally reached the Johnson cabin at the "head o' the holler." Slithering up the bank and clinging to the trees, I finally made it, using both hands to propel myself. How Diz got there, I'll never know, since she had her hands full of nursing bags, with none left over for clutching trees.

Edna's cabin is crowded, dirty and primitive. She is due now to bear her seventh baby. The others are shy, attractive towheads, the oldest not more than eight. Edna is probably twenty-five or younger, looking closer to forty-five. There is not a sign of a man-ufactured toy around the house, but the children appear to be happy and occupied.

The oldest girl is playing "dolls." She expertly rolls up a flour sack, ties a bit of rag around the neck, and tucks the doll into another flour sack cover for a bed. The range of play through which she puts this quickly-created doll is as wide as that of a city bred youngster with an expensive one—and just as imaginative.

She dresses her, puts her to bed, hauls her up and feeds her. Tiring of her, she unties the ragged ribbon, puts it on the shelf, and smooths the flour sack back into place with a pile of others. Diz is ready to examine Edna. At the mother's quiet request, "Young 'uns, go play outside," they cavort outdoors and are thereafter occupied with chasing chickens.

On a night, any time now, when Edna goes into labor, her hus-band will come for the nurses. They discuss the problem of getting the heavy delivery bags over the trail which we have covered. A horse could make it easily, but to reach this road from Hyden it is necessary to travel a couple of miles along the highway. Since the highway is pretty hard on the horses because of the pace of coal trucks (and hard on the student midwives, some of whom, like me, have only recently learned to ride), it is decided that they will come by Jeep to the point where the trail and highway meet and that Edna's husband is to bring the mule down to carry the bags from that point on.

Rarely, on these occasions where the nurse must go on foot, does she have to worry about transportation of her bags. If there is no mule, the husband (used to carrying hundred-pound sacks of flour up the creek) will meet her and pack her saddle bags. The families are exceedingly cooperative for the Frontier Nurses' care.

We finished at the Johnsons' and went on to Helen's, just around the bend. Helen had her baby several weeks ago, in the one-room cabin where we visited her. It had been Diz's first delivery in the district, so she showed Helen off with special pride.

A store-bought iron stove stood in the center for cooking and heating, and two old-fashioned brass bedsteads accommodated the baby's parents and his older brother. There was no separate crib; the baby was tucked under a flap of blanket in his parents' bed.

I looked in vain for an outhouse. The lack of one in the home of an older family would not have impressed me nearly as much. But this cabin was new and very carefully built, with considerable attention given to conveniences.

"Lots of these families still don't have a privy," Diz said. "We talk about it and give them building plans, but though they have to worm their youngsters regularly and get routine typhoid shots, they still can't seem to understand the need for sanitation."

We climbed back along the muddy trail, visited another patient, and were picked up on the highway and Jeeped back to supper.

December 15. The Log Cabin, as it is known, is a two-room structure, with a porch and bathroom, and hot water (if you want to fire up the temperamental little pot-bellied stove). It is perched on the side of the mountain overlooking Middle Fork and the ridge across the river.

Even in this season of mud and barren mountains, it is completely peaceful. In my room, a coal fire glows in the primitive stone fireplace. It is lovely and warm within a six-foot radius, freezing beyond that.

In Betty Lester's room, it is warmer, as she gets a certain amount of benefit when the bathroom stove is heated up. And though it means more work than coal, Betty is strictly a log fire advocate. Her room is lined with books. They—and Bruno, her dog—reflect the glow of firelight at any hour of the day or night and present the most restful surroundings I have ever known in which to talk, or read, or think, or just relax and go completely blank.

Betty is appointed official guide and interpreter of the Service during my visit here. In this particular, I've had a splendid break. She has been with the F.N.S. since 1928, interrupting her years here with seven spent in England from the outbreak of the war in 1939 until 1946.

During that time she served in a variety of jobs that brought her entirely up to date on midwifery trends. She loves and is devoted to the Service but her first two loyalties are much more basic: initially, to the whole program of maternal care in rural areas, and, secondly, to the mountain people of her adopted region. She has delivered hundreds of babies here. (Mrs. Breckenridge says thousands. Betty disputes the statement, though she has never kept score.) She knows every family in the area, and they are her friends.

Neither Betty nor Brownie, Mrs. Breckenridge's other assistant, had any theoretical preparation for her job. Both are exceptional teachers and have considerable administrative ability. They are more than adequately supplied with a natural gift for getting on with people and express themselves well. Brownie has a particularly rich vocabulary, with an imaginative choice of words and phrases.

Both read a great deal: professional and general literature. Betty would probably be an effective public speaker. Certainly, as we sit in front of the fire and talk about the F.N.S., she gets me so excited about the future of nurse-midwifery in America that I want to reach for an application blank for the Frontier Nursing School. Nevertheless, they are both so bound by the program of the F.N.S. that they do overlook many of the possibilities of making it a teaching service.

There is a good deal left to the individual initiative of the district nurse here. All of those who, even without theoretical preparation in public health, have a grasp of principles and of the possibilities of meeting needs within their districts are doing a thoroughly good job. But there are some, excellent bedside nurses and midwives though they be, who simply don't know public health as anything but giving shots.

Even on this limited basis, a considerable amount of credit is due. No immunization of any sort was available in the area before the Frontier Nursing Service came. Since then, immunization against typhoid, diphtheria, whooping cough and tetanus, and assorted other ailments has been given to a total of more than 165,000 shots. But there is one less than positive aspect of the service. The State of Kentucky lacks a strong public health program in the area. Therefore, the district nurses have taken the responsibility (which may have been forced upon them, true enough) for all health services.

As long as this situation goes along unchanged and nurses without public health preparation are used in the districts, F.N.S. itself is acting as a barrier between the mountain families and their possibilities of planning for improvement of their own health and welfare.

December 24. At Christmas the family feeling here at Wendover reaches high-water level and beneath the trees are hundreds of gaily decorated packages. Everybody remembers everybody. Gifts are usually jokes—with jingles. Bought things are frowned upon and considerable premium is placed upon ingenuity.

On Christmas Eve, the hospital nurses come from Hyden. There is something about people riding half a dozen miles on horseback across a swollen river to gather at a simple party. It's so out of keeping with the commercialized sort of Christmas. But then so are all the related festivities here: the simple service in the small log Chapel, the traditional employees' dinner at which all who ordinarily sit at the Big House table cook and serve a splendid feast, while all who ordinarily come in to work in the kitchen, laundry, barn, and gardens, sit at the Big House table.

Russie, the new and thoroughly frightened little girl from the "holler yonder down past Flat Creek" has been here just a scant three weeks. She watches the cook ring Mrs. Breckenridge's bell for service from the kitchen and as the whole twenty-nine "new" employees rush out with second helpings, Russie's timidity vanishes and she throws back her head and laughs; her homesickness is done with.

After dinner, Mrs. Breckenridge, with an actress's sense of timing (and a splendid voice for in-front-of-a-fire reading), marks this, as all special occasions, with a story, or with poetry read aloud. She chooses the "Seven Miracles of Gubbio" tonight, a lovely story built upon the St. Francis legend.

Christmas Day. We were up at the crack of dawn for a gorgeous winter sunrise. It had frosted during the night and every tree on the mountainsides was covered with an ethereal lacy icecoat. The sun rose almost scarlet and sent fluffy, rose-colored clouds across the sky. For perhaps half an hour, before the ice began to melt, the mountains were entirely pink and coral.

Joan and Stevie, the British nurses at the Flat Creek Center, had invited Mary (a Social Service worker), Hilly (a new nurse from England) and me to come for Christmas dinner. Leo, the Social Service Jeep, was scheduled for the trip and we took off early, dressed for the holiday in blouses, skirts and saddle shoes, instead of the usual jeans and boots.

We stopped at the Center on Red Bird River to pick up the nurses there. By this time the sun was high, and the frozen mud on the trail was melting quickly. Would we get across the river in the Jeep?

Mary said yes; Minnie, the nurse from Red Bird, did not think so. On we went in separate Jeeps, we and the giant shaggy Bruno in the front one, Minnie, Owen, and their dog Buddie in the second. Average speed: four miles an hour. Roads: washed out in spots and mud to the hubs in others.

Came the river: flowing fast and high. Consultation: "Yes" or "No?"

Mary: "Yes."

Minnie: "No."

Minnie: "Go ahead and try it, then."

Mary: "Are you game to try?"

We (starved by now and practically in sight of Christmas dinner): "Sure."

PLOP—Leo the Jeep starts across the river. Bruno the dog begins to howl mournfully. We reach the middle of the liver. Leo sputters.

We reach the high-water mark: two-thirds across. Leo stops, bogs down, and starts again. Mary's spine is a straight line, up and down.

We almost make the other side. Leo coughs and dies completely. Minnie stands on the bank, a definitely "I-told-youso" expression on her face. We try to divert Mary so she won't look back and see it, not on Christmas.

We remove our shoes and socks. "Should have worn boots," we mutter sadly. We open the door and the river flows through. We get out. The water is numbingly cold, the bottom horribly squishy. We push the Jeep. It rolls. Bruno leaps out and frolics in the water, splashing muddy river to our eyebrows. "Bruno," we shriek and, pleased, he leaps again. We push some more. Minnie yells across the water. Buddie barks. "Merry Christmas." Hmm !

Leo gets ashore. We relax.

Mary tries to start the Jeep. The spark plugs are full of river. We throw back the hood and stuff in Kleenex. The mud is ankle deep and soft and cold. We put on our shoes and socks. No use. The shoes remain embedded in the mud at every step. We take them off again. Our feet are blue beneath the coat of mud. "Merry Christmas."

We find a boat, or reasonable facsimile thereof. It is a raft of four wide planks and Mary poles it back across the river, using a sapling to guide it with. It's the funniest sight: grown women balancing on that tiny raft, and Bruno, in ecstasy at the prospect of being reunited with Buddie, leaping up and down and practically overturning it.

As the raft dwellers shout, "Stop him!", Bruno takes off on a one-dog committee of welcome, leaping upon his playmate. A sudden tangle of arms and legs and heads and fur and mud scramble onto the river bank as all of us are united.

We flounder back on the raft to Leo, where the Kleenex has successfully reconditioned every spark plug.

At the Flat Creek Center, Stevie and Joan took a single horrified look and silently brought out stacks of clothing. They piled neat stacks of wash cloths, soap and towels before us.

And eventually we all sat down to Christmas dinner. All of us, even Buddie and Bruno, sat and ate and slept. And Joan, who had never cooked a meal for company before, said we were wonderful house guests, appreciative of every detail.

December 30. "Doris," says Brownie at the table, "I've put you on call for all deliveries in the Hyden district. Most can be reached by Jeep or foot. And they'll phone here, every time a call comes in."

One comes at 6:30 the following morning and I race to Hyden. It's a premature call but the nurse decides to stay. Perhaps she'll come along faster than one would expect and there's not much point in returning home for a couple of hours.

The patient is eighteen and having her second baby. She is a thoroughly intelligent and cooperative mother, the wife of a local miner. Though early marriage interrupted her schooling, she is well-informed, well-read and considerably more sophisticated than most of the registered prenatal patients. Her home is modern, clean and comfortable, though sparsely furnished. A coal stove warms the place.

When we arrive, her pains are widely spaced and weak. She called early because her husband was away, her mother and sister working until noon, and she hesitated to remain alone, "in case it hurried." I was introduced as a District Nurse from New York, and throughout her labor there was never a minute when she was not the cordial hostess, trying to make me feel welcome. A student midwife, Ivy, was to do the delivery, and under Eva's supervision examined her patient and settled down to wait.

The patient, Mrs. Lewis, might have been serving tea to casual visitors during the first stage of her labor. We talked about her youngster (two years old) and her first delivery, which according to her statement was "nice and easy." We talked about Kentucky schooling, road building, miners' strikes.

The strikes were very hard on the miners' families. Mr. Lewis was a union miner in a nearby county. The union pay was considerably higher than the Leslie County workers got, but he had to board away from home, returning only on weekends. On a three-day work week this meant more out-go than income.

The Lewises were facing an acute disaster economically. Barbara, the two-year-old, was at a relative's until the baby came. "We gave her a doll for Christmas," her mother told us. "It's the first big one she ever had. Seemed as if she needed a baby to satisfy her, if I had one." While we talked the mother tended the coal stove, got out the blankets and clothing for the baby and put them on a chair by the fire to warm. She made a pot of coffee for the nurses, and got bathed and ready as her contractions were getting closer. Her interest in the whole phenomenon of birth was that of an alert spectator at a fascinating event of considerable importance to the group on hand.

She rested, she talked, she planned for the immediate future. We considered the relative merits of delivery in the hospital and home. Throughout this time the relationship between the student midwife and her patient was a constantly evolving interdependence on each other. Each was bringing out traits of courtesy and thoughtfulness in her companion. There was a feeling of deep peace inside the house.

The patient's sister brought little Barbara and her own new infant in for a couple of minutes' visit. Both women were casual and easy with the children, interested and relaxed about the progress of the labor. Helen, the sister, reminded Eva of the details of her own delivery which Eva had attended. Eva beamed with pleasure over the progress of that baby.

The visitors left. It was time to set up for delivery. Up to this point, some thirty minutes before the infant's birth, the mother had not given a single indication of physical discomfort except by a momentary change of expression during a contraction. By now, she said, they were "hard" and she frequently caught her breath, but still made no audible sound.

The mother-to-be checked the coal supply and furnace, then went to bed. Ivy checked her progress carefully, supervised by Eva, her instructor. Now she caught at the edge of the mattress, convulsively at each contraction. She still carried on a pleasant conversation between them. Ivy scrubbed up, and I bustled back and forth with water for the nested basins, which fit so neatly in the saddle bags.

The edge of the mattress was no longer a sufficiently satisfactory spot to clutch at. I stood beside her and she squeezed my hands. Her grip was like a vise.

We kept on talking, all of us, quietly, pleasantly, the patient wholly cooperative and responding perfectly to orders:

"Push with this contraction." "Rest." No need to urge her to push as long as each contraction lasted; she was working in perfect rhythm with them. I thought of Dr. Dick Read's words about the intelligent and properly informed mother and the relationship to childbirth. This was it! Not an iota of fear, perfect confidence and a job to do.

"We can see your baby—push it out."

Grunting, sweating, gripping my hands till the bones crunched, she worked with those contractions. Ivy and Eva were encouraging her, gently, Ivy supporting the perineum carefully against a tear. The head was delivered skillfully, the patient following instructions in every detail. The rest of the baby was delivered and held up for the mother to see it. "Here's your son," the midwife said, and the mother's eyes lighted up.

"Little fellow, isn't he?" she said. "He looks like Johnny."

"Tiny pinprick," Ivy apologized, as she gave a hypodermic of pitocin.

"Prick all you like—I've done my job," said the new citizen's mother in a tone of satisfaction.

Placenta expressed, ergotrate given, cord cut, fundus held, baby's eyes attended to, baby oiled and dressed, mother bathed, and equipment cleaned and packed.

By now the grandmother had arrived and then the father. Much rejoicing; general agreement that the baby did look like Johnny. Barbara in to see her brother, out to get her dolly, looking at both, critically; obviously deciding in favor of the doll. Doesn't want to eat the lunch her grandma made. "Want to get in Mommy's bed."

"Here, I'll feed her," mommy says. The new baby is forty seven minutes old. The mother is entirely comfortable. She looks contentedly at her son, then leans across to pass the spoon to Barbara. Barbara licks it and waves it toward the flannel bundle.

"Dolly," she says with interest.

"No—*brother*, Barbara, brother Johnny Junior."

Barbara licks the spoon again. "Brother Donny Dunyour," she agrees.

In the course of ten years of nursing, I've seen any number of deliveries and done a lot of prenatal work. But never until I came to Leslie County have I stayed beside a woman from the beginning of labor until she's had her baby. You don't, in city hospitals. Mothers are admitted in the clinic or on a private floor and "prepped" by the admitting nurse. They're tossed onto an elevator on a stretcher and conveyed to a row of labor rooms, where there's always someone in attendance, although it may be a different person every hour.

January 2, 1950. There's a delivery imminent at the hospital so I stay and discover myself still there at 9 p.m.

Question: How does one get to Wendover from Hyden this late at night?

Answer (in my head): One walks! It's moonlight and there's less reason for fussing about a moonlight walk through mountains of Kentucky than through New York City.

Brownie telephones. "The river's up. You'll have to stay in Hyden or walk in over the swinging bridge." I'm full of all these extraordinary deliveries. I want to talk to Brownie and Betty. "I'll walk."

I reach the swinging bridge, cold and lonely. The walk in from the highway after dark seems twice as long. I'm thinking about the mothers and their expressions when those babies are held up before the cord is cut. I reach the middle of the bridge and suddenly look over at the river.

By day the Middle Fork is swift and cluttered and muddy. But tonight the sky is full of stars, piled close together. And thousands of them have spilled into the river. Not a sound or a soul for a mile in either direction—just water rushing underneath the bridge, with stars spilled in it.

I think of Red Hook back in Brooklyn, where mothers can all get prenatal care and hospital confinements, for free if necessary, in chromium and green delivery rooms, and I think of the route from my home to the prenatal clinic via the subway's Sea Beach Express during rush hour in the mornings. And I look at the stars again—

in the sky and in the Middle Fork—and I measure what happened in the last few days against all the deliveries I've previously watched.

I race up the Wendover road in the dark and run up the Log Cabin steps, and Brownie and Betty and Bruno are waiting in front of the fire and we grin at one another sheepishly. And Betty laughs and says to Brownie, "I knew it. I told you so."

And Brownie says, "Wait until you're sure."

And Bruno offers a grubby paw and thoughtful scrutiny, then stretches out before the fire as if to say, "There's no place like it." And I sit and think about the mothers and the midwives.

And I think about Red Hook, which is more fun than any place I know to work in.

And I say, "Until I came here I thought I had the most satisfying job in the whole field of public health nursing."

And Brownie laughs and says thoughtfully, "And now you know it's the second most satisfying job?"

And we put more logs on the fire and talk. We talk about the F.N.S.-covered territory and of how every mother in it registers for maternity care. Because there are still areas covered by "Granny" midwives, some intelligent and clean, others questionable, out-of-district mothers even arrange to move in with a district family in order to be assured of proper care during a delivery. Brownie and Betty name half a dozen families. "They've begged us to start another district there beyond Flat Creek," they say, "but the staff and the budget can't stretch everlastingly."

The nurses admire Mrs. Breckenridge for her initial courage and vision in setting up the enterprise and they never let the questioner forget it.

"You've seen the difficulty in reaching patients now? Imagine, if you can, what it was like when F.N.S. began. We were seventy miles from the nearest highway. There were no trucks or Jeeps in all of Leslie County. It took a week on horseback to make rounds to all the outpost centers. It sometimes took seventeen hours and three fresh horses to bring a doctor in when help was needed.

"Every stick of wood and furniture and other supplies for the outpost centers was carried by mule team from the railroad, and dragged up creek beds to the sites. And do you know, there is just one reason why midwifery and district nursing succeeded in these mountains, while attempts to improve education failed.

"From the first, it was possible for the nurses to live in comfort, in homes they could be proud of, with adequate clinic facilities. You could bring in outside women with ability and energy and let them devote that energy to nursing. When outside school teachers came to Leslie County, their energy was mostly spent surviving the discomforts of local housing and cultural patterns. They never had the chance to concentrate on teaching."

This is loyalty indeed, for frontier non-midwife nurses are paid $120 monthly and out of this they must pay their board. Registered nurses who are licensed midwives (district nurses) are paid $135 monthly. Ditto about the board. There is no insurance coverage (other than accident insurance), no Social Security, no pension plan. You can't ride a horse forever!

But when the stars spill into the Middle Fork at night and Bruno stretches before the fire in the cabin, and you've just seen a delivery completed in that atmosphere of perfect confidence, you want to. Maybe there are some things a paycheck never compensates for.

January 10. Invariably if a sick child is brought to clinic, the father "packs hit in his arms," the mother walking behind him on the trail. Neither parent ever seems to scold or do anything which might upset the child. This sometimes results in tragic—or funny—situations. While I was standing in the hospital clinic, a mountain father carried in a child. The youngster looked acutely ill. Father stated he had been "ailing" for several days and so he brought him to the clinic. It had been a walk of several miles over a couple of mountains. He carried the heavy youngster tenderly all the way.

The doctor said it was pneumonia and that the child required hospitalization. Both parents immediately explained this to him. (The child was probably three years old.) Then they said, "You like to stop here in the hospital till you're better?" The child cried and said no, he wanted to go home.

Both parents looked at the doctor as though that settled it. "He don't want to stop here." Only the most careful (and tactful) follow-up by the doctor and the clinic nurse persuaded them to leave him. It was beyond their ken that parents would deliberately force a child to do something against his wishes.

Another pre-schooler came in with his mother, a sturdy mountain girl. Clinic conversation revealed that the young gentleman had not yet been weaned and both clinic nurse and doctor expressed concern about this. Mama shrugged and said there wasn't anything that she could do about it. "I try to wean him every now and then, but it makes him mad and he throws rocks at me."

January 12. We make a postpartum visit to a youngster who delivered a couple of days ago. The family is known as unreliable and is always in some kind of trouble. Since our visit the day before, the grandmother has been visited by "the law" for selling bootleg liquor. Neighbors tell us the story excitedly. She's to go to jail for thirty days, "sentence declared suspended until such time as the Frontier Nurses say her daughter can get out of bed."

Chapter 5

The Cornell Navajo Field Health Program

In the 1950-51 academic year I had the good fortune to be awarded a Rockefeller Foundation fellowship for advanced study in international health nursing. This I undertook at the University of Toronto, where an international program in public health and nursing administration had been developed.

This fellowship was in preparation for a position to teach public health nursing in Iran on the faculty of a new university school in Shariz, which would open in the fall of 1951.

At Toronto I took courses in epidemiology, public health and nursing administration. I delved into the literature of international nursing—which was new to me—and devoured all that I could read that would prepare me for this assignment.

At the close of the academic year, as I was ready to board ship for the Middle East, the plan was suddenly shattered by the flare-up of Anglo-American oil disputes. That resulted in British and American workers being barred from Iran for a considerable time.

It also delayed the opening of the new medical center and the university schools.

I had already been reassigned from the Visiting Nurse Association and was prepared to undertake public health nursing in a developing country. In despair, I sought the counsel of a nursing leader I admired, Virginia Dunbar, who was Dean of Cornell University-New York Hospital School of Nursing and Director of Nursing at the New York Hospital-Cornell Medical Center.

I described to her my experience, preparation and goals for teaching through example and demonstration in the clinical field. I reported sadly on the unexpected obstacle which had arisen and explained how much I wanted to bring public health nursing into an area of Iran that was without it.

"Miss Dunbar," I asked, "Do you know any place where there might be a similar opportunity, where there would be a chance to start from scratch in introducing public health nursing concepts and practices while the effect on the people's health could be measured?"

Miss Dunbar thought quietly for a moment or two. "Yes," she said. "I know the very spot. No public health nurse has ever worked there, and a totally new program of comprehensive family care is about to begin in a teaching setting, but without a public health nurse."

"Where, Miss Dunbar, where?" I asked eagerly.

She looked at me with some amusement.

"On the third floor of this building, in the General Medical Clinic. It would be a perfect opportunity to introduce the concepts of public health nursing to a teaching medical center. And here in our own country."

So I started to work in the Cornell Medical College's Comprehensive Care and Teaching Program, as a staff nurse in the

General Medical Clinic, and on the Monday following my inter-
view with Dean Dunbar. Some forty years later I now cheerfully
confess that I had a hidden agenda of introducing the principles
and practice of public health nursing into the clinic's daily routine.
If I gave any thought to an anticipated time-frame I suppose it was
in terms of the three-year period which I had agreed to spend in
Iran. I remained at Cornell in one patient-care-centered program or
another for the next twenty-nine years, in a series of extraordinarily innovative nursing opportunities.

One of these was on the Navajo Indian reservation in Arizona.
Dr. Walsh McDermott, the Livingston Farrand Professor of Public
Health at Cornell Medical College, and one of the discoverers of
izoniazid, had carried out studies of the drug's effect on hospitalized tuberculosis patients there. The drug, in combination with
others, proved effective and Dr. McDermott turned his attention to
intervening in the disease process itself. Among the semi-migrato-
ry Navajo sheepherders, the patterns of health and disease could
be observed in relation to day-by-day community life.

This was still a primitive culture living in relative isolation. Up
to now the caretaking Anglo society and the 80,000 rural Navajos
were so different and so mutually misunderstood that the Bureau
of Indian Affairs' efforts to deliver health services to them had
been poorly accepted and were far less than effective. The wide-
spread tuberculosis and the measles epidemics on the reservation
attested to this.

Recognizing that there was a missing bridge between the white
doctors and nurses working on the reservation and their Navajo
patients, Dr. McDermott, with the assistance of Dr. Kurt Deuschle
and a fine anthropologist, Dr. John Adair, proposed to set up a
remote rural clinic at Manyfarms, a site selected by the tribe, and
there to train Navajo assistants to the public health nurses already
working on the reservation.

Three or four native "health visitors" could extend the work of one public health nurse to serve the rural population with more comprehensive as well as more acceptable care. The type of training and the degree to which the largely-unschooled Navajo students could be taught to extend the community's health care successfully was yet to be determined; experimentation and careful evaluation were necessary.

As with any new cross-cultural health project, there was movement in many directions all at once. Erecting a workable clinic at a barren desert site and providing housing for the professional and trainee workers and their families produced a series of decisions, tribal and medical, which were not always satisfactory. The clinic was set up and the first class already was in residence, for instance, before the on-site physician and public health nurse had had time to consider the Navajo assistants' curriculum.

Help was sought from the Cornell School of Nursing, and Dean Dunbar asked me to make the site visit to evaluate the situation.

June 27, 1955. I spent today in Albuquerque with the area consultant in nursing for Indian Services and found her friendly and outgoing but "troubled about the Cornell project." I listened a lot and said very little. She seems to be reacting in part with hurt feelings "because nursing was never in on the planning of this program."

The nursing consultant, together with the Bureau of Indian Affairs' doctors with whom she works, generally have expressed considerable anxiety over the use of Navajo health visitors. I ask about the specific hazard they are concerned with. The comments are vague and seem to stem from a fear of the unknown. There are remarks such as "pseudo-doctors, trained in a few weeks," and "unlicensed practice of medicine and nursing."

I visited the Indian school for practical nurses and the Indian T.B. sanatorium. The government service takes real pride in the operation of this school and in the practical nurses it graduates, who are later assigned to various Indian reservation hospitals. The school is attractive, well-equipped and staffed, and appears to have an excellent course of study.

Unfortunately, relatively few Navajo women apply and of those who do, many upon graduating ask to be assigned to a reservation other than their own. They've learned a different way of life from their families.

I find, to my regret, that to be eligible for admission, candidates must have completed a four-year high school course. A history of tuberculosis will disqualify an applicant, and each application must be accompanied by a letter "from the applicant's pastor."

Applicants truly representative of the rural Navajo are thus ineligible to become health workers. I begin to understand a bit more clearly Cornell's desire to develop the health visitor as a new kind of worker.

I flew across the desert to Gallup just at sunset; there were red-gold cliffs, miles of wasteland and endless space. A wonderful feeling of remoteness. It is a beautiful country.

June 28. I have met Bernice Laughlin, the Cornell project's public health nurse. She has had seven years of experience with the Indian Service on the reservation, good T.B. sanatorium experience, prior to that with Army service in Europe.

She picks me up in her car for a shopping expedition.

"You' re going to have to set up a trailer to live in. They're secondhand and not notably clean, so go buy yourself supplies for the next three weeks. Be sure to get yourself a broom and scouring powder...." With that she dropped me off at a Gallup supermarket for half an hour while she took off to have the car overhauled.

Having fixed up a hundred-year-old rural one-room school-house in Pennsylvania and a tenement apartment on York Avenue in New York, I considered half an hour not unreasonable.

"There's not a thing in it," shouts Bernie from the car, "not even a can opener." I shop frantically for pots and pans, canned goods, two plates, forks and knives, a couple of cups and saucers (must be equipped for a guest, of course) and dish towels.

"Anything you don't get now you'll have to do without for the next three weeks."

I invest in waxed paper, toilet paper, carrots, radishes, aluminum foil (equally good for wrapping sandwiches or making window curtains) and am on the curb with my bounty when the car pulls in.

We stop at Window Rock, the tribal headquarters, to meet the sub-area consultant in public health nursing, who had been Bernie's immediate supervisor prior to Bernie's transfer to the Cornell Project. I asked about their official relationship now and learned that while Bernie continues to send in a monthly report of her work (immunizations, home visits, etc.) to the department and to requisition supplies as they are needed, she is otherwise pretty isolated as far as nursing contacts go, and has no direct nursing supervision.

The consultant offers me the opportunity of seeing a good deal more, of the public health nursing activities on the reservation than the Cornell clinic, "in order to get the Manyfarms project in perspective." I am delighted to have the chance. Bernie seems delighted also; she will show me. No, the consultant will show me. They appear to be under some tension. Compromise: all three of us will take a weekend trip to Tuba City and points enroute, on the second weekend of my stay. Everybody seems satisfied with this.

June 29. The Cornell clinic and twelve trailers for personnel, bought from a defunct housing project, are set in a treeless, sun-baked stretch of ground on a reasonably good dirt road. Ditches around the whole encampment now contain hundreds of tiny deadlooking sticks, newly planted, which, if luck is with us, will presently grow into shade-giving Russian olive trees. The prospect for this seems dim at a glance; however, these trees do grow quickly. Bernie predicts that by September the appearance of the project will be greatly changed.

Everyone lives here "family style": the doctor and his wife, the public health nurse, the health visitors and other members of the staff, together with their families.

You feel their warmth and friendliness the minute you climb out of the car, and soon recognize that whatever may or may not be true about the health visitors' work performance, there are many exceptional values taking root here. There is humor and spontaneity in the welcome I receive and within minutes I feel a part of the group.

Jim Hitzrot, the doctor, and Bernie Laughlin are presently the only non-Navajo staff in residence. Within a few days Don Reader, the social scientist, is due to arrive. Bobbie, Jim's wife, makes a solid contribution to morale as she waits out the final weeks of her first pregnancy and extends herself in friendly fashion to the shy Navajo wives.

Jim is assuredly a first-rate choice. He is young, just through his internship (Princeton English major, Harvard Medical, and a year of internship at Hopkins). Has not yet begun his residency, which will be in orthopedics when his two-year service with the U.S. Public Health Service is completed. He is resourceful, eager, and a very sound skipper for the Navajo crew, which, with one exception, is composed entirely of ex-T.B. patients. There are laboratory and x-ray technicians and a clerk, as well as the health visitors.

This is the only place on the reservation where I've met such complete faith in the ability of the Navajos to prove themselves. Therein, I think, lies Cornell's (or more accurately, Doctors McDermott, Deuschle and Adair's) basic tenet, which differs so radically from the medical care programs traditionally offered here.

I reflect a bit on the why of traditional health education and recognize the importance of standards; licensure is one effective approach. But I think of how easy it is—in medicine or nursing or even grade-school teaching—to let tradition take over a curriculum and inure it against change. And how human are the reactions of inertia, fear of change and of new costs when any new educational approach is suggested to those with a vested interest in continuing the traditional.

I think, too, of that wonderful excerpt from John Collier about the Indians and his passionate belief in "making people free by helping them to confront real emergencies which they are capable of mastering." In that fragment of a sentence, it seems to me, lies the entire philosophy of the Cornell-Navajo Field Health Project. The testing of that hypothesis I believe to be important research as truly as the diarrhea study or the T.B. home care experiment are research.

If it is true that the preparation of health visitors in an experimental program is a research study, then, like any thoughtful study, there must be set down a hypothesis and evidence as it accumulates in order that the final conclusions be made by evaluating systematically recorded observations. This has not been done and, I think, represents the one area in which the government people have a logical point in their objections to this pioneer program.

July 7. I'm writing this from my trailer, set out in the desert behind the prefab tin building which is the Cornell clinic. We're located on a wide plateau in the geographical center of the vast desert, where the wind blows sizeable dust storms daily but where the view is magnificent whenever it isn't blowing. After dark a million bright stars are so close that you can almost touch them.

In every direction native hogans are visible, if one looks for them carefully. They blend so well with the clay-colored plateau that at first one has the impression that there can't be any Indians here.

But, at 8 a.m., when the clinic opens, the Indians appear from somewhere; on foot, in horse-drawn springless wagons, and in the back of rickety pick-up trucks. There are old men with long hair and handkerchiefs around their heads, huge hunks of turquoise in their ears; grandmothers in velvet blouses trimmed with coins and silver buttons; cradle-boarded babies tightly bound hand and foot in swaddling clothes of worn-out flour sacks; and school children in T-shirts and blue jeans.

The clinic is about 75 miles northwest of Fort Defiance, 110 miles from Gallup. These clinic patients are primarily from the families of sheepherders; they are generally far less sophisticated than the Fort Defiance Indian families, yet even here there is great variation in living standards, from primitive to considerably comfortable.

July 11. Today I got a look at the local trading post in the valley, which has only Navajo clientele. It carries the most essential staples: sugar, salt, condensed milk, coffee, a sprinkling of such canned goods as pork and beans, and heavy hardware such as galvanized-iron water barrels and laundry tubs. Gallup is the source of uncanned fruits and vegetables, and just about anything else in the way of supplies. I was entranced to see among the indispensables the trading post carries is a sizeable stock of toy cap pistols and rolls of 1000 loud-popping caps.

Cowboys and Indians even here?

Yes, it's true; the Navajo health visitor in the trailer next to mine has a wonderfully amusing six-year-old, Vernon, with two passions in life: baseball and Indians. He visits my trailer and leafs through copies of the *Saturday Evening Post* to point out pictures of his heroes in both categories. Indians, to him, are strictly limited to the feathered and war-painted variety worshiped by any New York kid. I inquire casually if he isn't an Indian too and Vernon looks at me as though I'm not too bright. "I *play* I'm an Indian but I'm really a Navajo," he says.

July 16. Bernie runs a Girl Scout troop in Gallup, to which she drives 110 miles each way for weekly meetings. She asked if I would be willing to help her troop earn money for summer camp by joining them, last Saturday night, in selling hot dogs at the semiannual used-truck auction held in Gallup. This, I was told, was an opportunity, par excellence, to observe the Indian family adapt to culture change. The used-truck auctions are social as well as business events, with families traveling up to a hundred miles by horse and wagon to bid on one of the 80 or 90 auctioned trucks.

I watched from the vantage point of the hot-dog stand at least 200 Indians bidding frantically—and I opened more than 800 bottles of Coke while observing Navajos-in-action. Having piled up these profits of exploitation on behalf of the Gallup Girl Scouts, I returned somewhat shamefacedly to the clinic, there to extol the nutritional and budgetary advantages of powdered skim milk, in my regular capacity as visiting instructor to the Navajo health visitors.

July 19. I had the opportunity to sit in on the Tribal Council's monthly Health Committee meeting, an experience I wouldn't have missed for anything. One is impressed by the warmth of feeling which the tribal delegates have for "Dr. McDermick's" program, although plenty of education will be needed before most of them really understand either the goals or methods of it.

July 20. All the Indian staff members have recently learned to drive and they are enormously proud of this accomplishment. They are proud also of the sturdy sky-blue Cornell station wagons. They exhibit these with much the same affection which their ancestors had for horses—and they ride them not too differently! Even a "good" reservation road is a pretty indifferent specimen, and en route to outlying hogans one uses wagon trails or simply takes off across the sandy desert floor.

Today Frank, an enormously tall and heavy student health visitor, apprenticed to a medicine man prior to developing T.B., and now the most earnest and ambitious of the students, invites me to supervise his first group of hogan visits. (Since the students are far more at ease with Bernie, who has been their teacher, she makes the usual supervisory nursing visit with them in the field.) I am delighted to be asked, and Frank and I settle down with the patients' charts.

The first home visit involves checking on a baby seen a day earlier in the clinic and treated there for diarrhea. The mother failed to return with her and we plan to visit for three reasons:

(1) To see how the youngster is responding to treatment and, if indicated, to continue the therapy ordered by the doctor.

(2) To ascertain whether the mother's failure to return is due to the child's improvement (she must carry her several

miles in the scorching sun and may rightly have decided that the benefits of another visit would be outweighed by the difficulties), or whether we, in the clinic, had failed to meet her expectations and her failure to return was the result of disillusionment. (In these first few weeks of running the clinic service this is a must to check on, for delivery of health care across a cultural barrier is dependent on establishing and maintaining good rapport.)

(3) To take a second specimen (rectal swab) from the baby for the infant diarrhea study.

Frank gallops the station wagon over the desert. (Dr. McDermott is having the cars equipped with seat belts. No explanation is required after one has gone home-visiting with Frank.)

We reach the hogan and go inside. Like the majority of older hogans in the district, this is a six-sided log structure, heavily encased with mud for insulation. The mud makes it delightfully cool but very dark inside. In the center stands an efficient homemade oil can stove, its chimney of soldered tin cans extending through the smoke hole in the roof.

The family's blankets, goatskins, and clothing are neatly hung on wall pegs; an old kitchen cabinet and a pedal-operated sewing machine are the only manufactured articles of furniture. The mother is sewing. The baby is laced in a cradle board and propped-up nearby, looking far more chipper and less dehydrated than she had a day earlier in clinic.

Greetings are exchanged in Navajo and Frank reminds the mother that I am the nurse she met earlier. He explains the purpose of our visit and the mother reports her daughter much improved. She plans to return on Saturday when her husband comes from planting corn and their horse and wagon is available.

Frank asks permission to take the baby's temperature and the rectal swab. The mother takes a shaggy goatskin from the wall and spreads its furry surface on the earthen floor. Kneeling, she unlaces the baby from her cradle board and puts the naked six-week-old in the center of this temporary rug.

Since Frank and I are fairly tall, the problem of flipping this tiny mite on her tummy and obtaining the swab can only be solved by getting closer to her. We kneel on either side of the goatskin. Frank turns the baby over and opens the sterile swabs. I take out a match and flame the culture-media container. Frank inoculates it and then, since there is no adequate way of disposing of the contaminated swab safely, I light another match, we ignite the swab and solemnly kneel there while it burns the length of the wooden stick in Frank's uplifted hand.

Suddenly, kneeling there, I remember the Kluckholm documentary film on the ceremonies of the Navajo medicine man which Dr. McDermott has shown to the medical students: the dying infant, the sand paintings on the hogan floor, the ceremonial chants, the thousand years of folklore bringing comfort to the family. And I realize in a flash that Frank and I are going through a ceremony which could be dubbed right into that documentary.

I look at the mother; she watches us closely and apparently with satisfaction. Frank removes the thermometer and hisses softly to the baby the Navajos' "Sss-Sss-Sss," which parents use as a lullaby or expression of endearment in the clinic waiting room.

I get to my feet with a considerable creak. The mother replaces the baby in her cradle board and puts the goatskin on the wall. We say good-bye. I look behind me as we climb into the station wagon and I wonder: "Cornell—replacing superstition with scientific medicine?" Frank wonders a little too, as we charge across the desert, and between that hogan and the next one he sings me the part he knows of the "sing" for a sick child, the "Navajo Blessing Way."

I ask Frank how much a "sing" helps and he looks thoughtful. "Many times, very much," he reports. "I had three sings when I was sick. First two, I felt a lot better for a long while. Last one I didn't. Then I went and got an X-ray. That time the doctor showed me a T.B. germ in the microscope; that's when I decided to go back and teach my people. For some things the medicine man, for some things the doctor. Most Navajo go to the doctor when the medicine man fails. Now, maybe we can get the doctor and the medicine man to work together."

At the Manyfarms clinic it looks as though that may be going to happen. Walsh McDermott, and his friend Dan Yassi, a powerful tribal medicine man, dedicated the clinic jointly. Each respected and understood the other, each admitted his limitation in understanding the other's work and each had a similar goal for the community: preventing untimely death and needless suffering.

July 28. Frank and Ruth are products of the first health visitors' class. I have gone over Bernie's lesson notes, observed Ruth and Frank in clinic, watched their interaction with patients as well as their techniques, and each night checked their entries in the charts of patients seen that day. What I see and hear, with a few exceptions, is encouraging.

These workers are already skilled in simple techniques and show a real flair for teaching. Their approach is remarkably comprehensive, showing concern with a range of problems rather than one single factor.

Last February both Ruth and Frank were almost without the ability to write English, although they spoke it fluently. They are still exceedingly limited in this skill. Yet bound by this limitation, they are managing to recognize the essentials in any given situation, act upon this recognition, and record the work done and plan for the future concisely and with judgment.

Here is an entry made by Ruth on a patient's record:

"She had little baby girl at home four days ago. She had not enough milk for baby. She just ate bread and coffee. I told her, drink lots of milk, eat some vegetable and meat. Could she bring baby back tomorrow?"

When Ruth made her first hogan visit it was to a mother recently released from the sanatorium to plan for returning the mother's baby (born during her T.B. hospitalization) from its present foster care. Before the visit Bernie discussed with Ruth the reasons why a pre-discharge call was made to the home, the importance of noting the environment into which the baby would be coming, the need for appraising the mother's ability to give care, and her attitude toward the baby's return.

All this, said Bernie, would be of interest to the social worker at Gallup who counted on us for this information. As a matter of fact, Bernie added, perhaps Ruth would like to write the letter to the social worker after making the hogan visit.

Ruth's letter read as follows:

"Manyfarms Clinic

June 7, 1956

"Dear Robinson *Ruth wastes no ink on titles,*

"I just want to tell you about Rose Ann Tsosie. We went visit her home yesterday we told her they bring her baby back to her June 26.

"She had nice clean home she keep everything clean her food and drink water and dishes all covered. We told her how she going to take care of that baby. Not to let him go near any sick person why we telling her this because baby now is well. We told her they take good care of him at St. John. She says she be glad to get her baby back soon too.

...This will be for now."

Frank's notes are briefer but equally broad in coverage and like most of Frank's reasoning, utterly logical.

"6/5/56 We visit Bessie Claw to tell her about—
1)   Blood test
2)   To clinic for medicine—return
3)   Plan to get X-ray
4)   Skin test of children

"Arrangements made for her to take Children to Ft. Defiance Thursday 6/8/56 for X-rays-Skin Test
"6/9/56 Bessie Claw went."

One more example of Frank's reports:

"6/5/56-Visit Keith Curly's family

"We find out
1)   Keith to work
2)   Wife of Keith under medical care
3)   Baby got X-ray
4)   Keith's mother got X-ray
5)   Mary Shorty want X-ray
6)   Joe Shorty will go for X-ray too."

Both Frank and Ruth will need careful supervision in the weeks ahead to help them develop their strengths (accuracy and range of observation, future plans, etc.) and to help them recognize weak areas: listing dosages and instructions given with medications, insuring that all the important pieces of history are written down, and above all, from a legal point of view, that the signature of the doctor ordering a medicine or treatment in the clinic is added to the chart.

I doubt that many young doctors with Jim's one year of internship behind him would have been likely to recognize the hazard of health visitors acting without signed orders. Bernie, for her part, said that in these initial weeks of establishing a clinic routine she had been divided in her feelings. On the one hand, the use of unsigned orders did indeed leave the health visitors uncovered and unaware of their responsibilities, but on the other hand she wanted very much not to appear an obstructionist, "as full of red tape as a government supervisor."

Jim, Bernie, and I talked over the need for standing orders, which the trainees would follow specifically when they did not have written orders for treatment of patients. In hospitals such safeguards are taken care of by administrative committees, prodded by the hospital and nursing school licensure inspectors.

Standing orders might cover: routine nursing care; simple nursing procedures such as alcohol sponge, hot packs, enemata; medication orders under specific circumstances, including exact dosage, i.e., in case of penicillin reaction, or other adverse circumstances; routine immunization procedures; and First Aid.

I suggested that in the clinic, orders for treatment or medication be written on the record by the physician (or by the health visitor) and be signed by the physician before they are carried out and that this be considered a "must" by the health visitors. A tape-recorded commentary by Bernice and the health visitors offers the only actual record available to document this first class's learning and progress.

As a record of growth it is a first-rate project. As a way of evaluating the student's learning, its usefulness will be more limited; one has only their own conviction that "we learned a lot," which they undoubtedly did.

Before the start of a new class I would like to see a curriculum written up in a fairly definite fashion, even though its content remains elastic, and the entire curriculum be subject to radical change before the third group arrives.

August 12. In the middle of the desert, in northern Arizona, in the heart of the Navajo country, I am witnessing an example of the ultra-fashionable technique of role playing, the more effective because no one thinks of or recognizes it as anything special. "Skills," Jim and Bernie will tell you, "the Navajo visitors learn in record time. The problem is their embarrassment over asking questions, their difficulty with vocabulary, and their reluctance to admit their inability to understand or to cope with a complex situation."

To overcome this diffidence, Jim and Bernie have instituted as permissive a classroom and clinic atmosphere as possible, but even in this setting Frank and Ruth and Deswood (another student visitor) find it hard to say, "I don't understand." To test their comprehension and to provide an additional teaching tool, Jim created a fictitious character: "The old man from Navajo Mountain."

Navajo Mountain is an almost inaccessible piece of land in the northwest corner of the reservation, an area which still harbors Indians who have never made face-to-face contact with a white man. The vast majority of the Navajo live a primitive life, but most are familiar with a rather wide range of modern technological developments. Most families, for example, own a radio and pedal sewing machine. Most Navajo have ridden in a truck. Even in the most outlying trading post, most understand the workings of an automatic Coke machine. But to the Navajo who are master of this knowledge, the native of Navajo Mountain is the symbol of an earlier era, a hillbilly, whose lack of sophistication makes him the target of their humor.

Thus, when Ruth and Frank had learned the technique of giving an immunization injection and could repeat the explanation of its action knowledgeably, Jim or Bernie would further test their comprehension of the principle involved and their ability to adapt an explanation to the hearer's level, by saying, "That's fine."

"Now, instead of explaining it to a mother who has come to clinic, suppose you've gone into the mother's hogan to give the baby's shot. When you get there, the baby's grandfather is home. He's just come down from Navajo Mountain to live with them. He doesn't trust injections. How are you going to tell him what it's for?"

By this device, the old man from Navajo Mountain has drawn out the student's knowledge and introduced an additional problem to be solved, that of communication. Since custom permits Jim and Bernie, as well as the health visitors, to view "the old man" with humor, this lightens the atmosphere of the classroom and permits the students to tackle the harder tasks with less tension.

Unexpectedly, the students themselves took over the old man from Navajo Mountain. Quick to seize on the pretense element as a way they could save face but still acquire knowledge, they, rather than Jim and Bernie, continued to produce him in classroom and clinic situations. Faced with a fact which they could not fully comprehend, one or the other health visitor would solemnly say, "Dr.

Hitzrot," (or "Miss Laughlin,") "How would you tell that to the old man from Navajo Mountain?" Then, digesting the simplified explanation, they'd be ready to move on.

Jim and Bernie and I were delighted, of course, for the old man's fictitious presence permitted the visitors to be far more honest about admitting their own academic limitations.

"Now tell that to the old man from Navajo Mountain," was a daily classroom challenge. Sometimes the old man turned up at lunch or in odd off-hours to show that the formal curriculum carried over even to these times.

We were scattered throughout the empty clinic yesterday morning, checking supplies. Deswood was cleaning the laboratory, Ruth preparing bundles for the autoclave, and Frank unpacking instruments. Suddenly, over the partitions came Deswood's anguished voice:

"Dr. Hitzrot! Old man from Navajo Mountain's in the lab. Won't let me stick him for a blood count. How do I explain it to him?"

Jim, whose sense of the dramatic is only a short lap behind his ability as a physician, rose to the occasion. "Charley, Ruth, Frank, all the staff," he shouted, "get to the lab quickly! Old man from Navajo Mountain's got Des down. Help him!" Laughing, everybody scrambled into the empty lab where Deswood sat labeling slides.

"Ruth, you help Des," said Jim. "What could you tell the old man about that blood count?"

One by one various explanations were offered and pulled apart by the group until finally one was synthesized to everyone's satisfaction. Then we all got back to work.

Once a Navajo woman came into the clinic with a history that made the diagnosis of incomplete abortion probable. Now our health visitors are amazingly knowledgeable, but when a situation arises in which their traditional cultural pattern runs counter to their newfound knowledge, they are still in a very uncomfortable spot.

This was such an occasion. So rudimentary is the migratory Navajo's concept of anatomy and physiology that all organs below the diaphragm are usually called by a single term. Thus, understandably, the rationale behind a pelvic examination is difficult to explain, and this procedure, which has only a sexual connotation, is one for which it is very hard to obtain consent.

Jim explained to Ruth what the patient's physical problem was and what he wanted to do. Ruth nodded, accepting the explanation, yet obviously she was reluctant to interpret this to the waiting patient.

Bernie realized that Ruth was caught between the two cultures' ways of thought and she sat down with her for about twenty minutes to review the patient's needs and the function of health workers in meeting these needs. At first Ruth identified entirely with the woman—overidentified, in fact. So sure was she that the patient would never accept a pelvic examination that she was unable to find Navajo words to explain the doctor's reason for wanting to do this.

Finally, coached minutely, she talked with the patient and, to her surprise, obtained consent rather easily. She draped the patient for the examination and called the doctor. Jim, who had heard her reluctant argument with Bernie, entered the cubicle. He complimented Ruth on how well she had handled the explanation, then added, teasingly, "Now, Ruth, this woman's father came in with her. He's from Navajo Mountain and he's out there in the waiting room. How are you going to explain this exam to him?"

Ruth looked utterly defeated. She was truly stunned by the thought. Three times she began a sentence in Navajo. Each time, after a reluctant syllable or two, she shook her head. Obviously that explanation would not do.

She worked this problem over for several minutes, then spun on her heel and looked Jim in the eye.

"Dr. Hitzrot," she said in a great rush of words, as though their pressure was intolerable, "Dr. Hitzrot, if I were you, I'd just do that examination before the old man comes in here!"

Dr. Hitzrot followed her advice. And Ruth looked mighty relieved when she discovered that the waiting room was empty.

"I didn't think Dr. Hitzrot meant the old man was real," she muttered. "But some day that old man from Navajo Mountain's gonna be there. And we better learn more than we know before he comes."

August 20. Nurses, physicians and other health workers often fail to recognize how much culture affects the way a patient and his family seek treatment and respond to medical personnel. Even in the absence of understanding, however, respect for the family's rights to their own beliefs can enable one to work comfortably and helpfully with another culture.

It may be easy to recognize the barriers to accepting medical care when one is working with a relatively isolated culture, such as the Navajo. On the cosmopolitan urban American scene, in New York City, say, it is often harder to determine the influence of culture on patients' behavior.

These two examples are from widely separated home-care problems, yet, despite the unique cultural perspective of each family, I discovered surprising similarities between them.

In a Navajo Hogan

Mary T. was a fifty-nine-year-old Navajo woman diagnosed as having an epidermoid carcinoma of the cervix. She was admitted to a private hospital for radiation therapy. From there she was transferred to a government (Indian) hospital and discharged a month later with a poor prognosis.

After discharge, she was followed in her home community by the Cornell-Navajo clinic. Here an additional diagnosis of osteoblastic carcinoma was made. She was re-hospitalized for ten days at a mission hospital, but her family wished to give her terminal care at home.

Family members came to the clinic to ask if the staff would help care for Mary after her discharge from the hospital. Jim re-explained the nature of her illness and told them there was no known cure for her condition at this time. The family replied that a Navajo medicine man had given them hope that Mary might be cured and they wanted to seize every opportunity.

The Navajo people do not distinguish between health and religious practices. They see health as a perfect balance between man and his environment, an environment that includes people, nature, and the supernatural. We would call this the natural, religious, and social surroundings of a patient.

The Navajo believe that illness means a person has fallen out of his delicate environmental balance and that health can be restored by the acts of a fellow man who has proper and exact knowledge of myth and ritual, namely, the medicine man.

Jim agreed with the family about using the "sings" of the medicine man, but asked that simultaneously (with the medicine man's approval) the Cornell clinic staff be permitted to extend whatever help the patient required and could accept.

Mary T. returned to her camp by horse and wagon. The camp consisted of two hogans and a sheep corral. One hogan was occupied by the patient and John T., her husband, the other by Mary's niece and the niece's husband. Several nephews, whom the patient had raised, lived in the camp from time to time.

Jean French, P.H.N., and Ruth, the health visitor, made bi-weekly visits to show the family how to nurse the patient and make her comfortable. When it seemed indicated, they gave Mary direct nursing care. The clinic provided medications, dressings, and necessary equipment.

John T. improvised a trapeze, at Jean's suggestion, so his wife could alter her position with less pain. Her back had become excoriated while she was hospitalized, and Jean taught the husband to give back care. He did this so effectively that he was able to halt the development of a decubitus ulcer. When Jean checked the supply of medicines on successive visits, however, it became plain that the family was not giving medicine as directed.

The health visitor believed that the family withheld the pills because they associated the patient's physical decline with the medicines which she had begun to take in the hospital and feared that more would make her worse. Jean made several visits while the patient was having a "sing." On occasions when a "sing" was interrupted by her visit, she was permitted to give care in the presence of the medicine man.

During the patient's downhill course, the family kept her as comfortable as possible and followed the staff's suggestion to maintain adequate fluid intake. Shortly before the patient's death, the family called in a native diagnostician, the *ni delnuhi,* who said that the patient would die at noon that day. The Navajo must bum the hogan in which someone dies, so the patient was moved to an expendable, temporary hogan made of logs and bushes, about 500 yards from the hogan in which she had lived.

Jean noticed that Mary seemed very cold, although she still responded to sound and movement. John T. had purchased two new woolen blankets and a satin comforter for Mary, and as she became progressively colder, Jean thought their use seemed indicated.

However, the family explained that these new blankets could be used only after death. For the first time, Jean found it difficult to accept the family's ways. By now, Mary was aphasic, her respirations shallow and rapid, but her pulse still strong.

On the following morning, family members came to the clinic to report that the patient was dying. Jim, Jean, and Ruth went out to the hogan and found Mary T.'s condition as it had been on the previous day. The family was taught how to check the patient's pulse and a small mirror was left with them to check her breathing. Later that day the family sent word that Mary had no pulse and that her breath no longer coated the mirror.

A hogan visit was made to confirm the fact of death. The immediate family and other relatives were gathered outside the temporary hogan. They asked Jean if she would prepare the patient for burial. The Navajo are afraid to touch a body after death, because they believe that the spirit or ghost of the departed person is contaminating.

Yet the family said that the two nephews could help and the patient's husband, John, went into the shelter to supervise the activities. It was unusual for a Navajo family to permit Navajos to touch a body, and they later arranged for a cleansing "sing" to counteract any contamination of the nephews.

When Jean had completed postmortem care, the husband asked her to dress his wife's body in her best squaw dress, with a long, satin, pleated skirt and a long-sleeved, velvet blouse trimmed with silver coins. A kerchief was put around her neck and her turquoise jewelry—ring, bracelet, and necklace—were put on her body. A clay resembling red ochre was given Jean to rub on Mary's face to give it a more natural appearance. Her hair was brushed, rolled, and put into a net.

Then John T. took all his money out of his wallet, put it into a little red purse, and had Jean put this on Mary's body. The squaw blanket was put on her, then the two new woolen blankets, and finally the new satin comforter.

Ruth had been in the temporary shelter all this time, but Jean was aware of her reluctance to touch the body and did not ask her to help with the procedure. The husband thanked Jean for her help and wept when he spoke of the fine woman that Mary T. had been. The family waited outside the hogan for a Christian missionary, who was to bring a wooden coffin and officiate at the burial service. Later that evening, the temporary hogan in which Mary had died was burned, in accordance with Navajo tradition.

In an Urban Tenement

Anthony F., a seventy-three-year-old, partly retired junk dealer, who was born in Italy but had lived most of his life in New York City, was discharged from the New York Hospital after a course of radiation therapy following a diagnosis of cancer of the bladder. He had refused consent for an operation, which the doctors thought essential. His several adult children were told of his poor prognosis. Anthony F.'s wife had recently been hospitalized with myocardial infarction, and was being cared for at home by the youngest daughter, Catherine, unmarried and aged twenty-four.

Since the nursing care of two seriously ill parents seemed more than this daughter could cope with, the hospital staff recommended a nursing home in the neighborhood for Anthony F. Both he and his family vigorously resisted the idea.

Six married sons and daughters and a widowed sister of his lived in the vicinity. They were willing to contribute to the financial support of the F. household and they declared that both parents could be adequately cared for by Catherine.

The home care nurse-coordinator and the social worker both tried to explain how heavy the burden of round-the-clock care would be, but the patients' sons were adamant. Catherine seemed fearful of the responsibility of caring for her father but willing to try. She was able to think about care at home on a tentative and possibly temporary basis.

Her brothers were not. So Anthony F. was taken home by ambulance, and the visiting nurse was asked to assess the family's need for assistance and to give what help was acceptable to them. Especially, she would teach Catherine such essential technical procedures as irrigation of her father's indwelling catheter and would help Catherine talk about her own problems.

When the visiting nurse first entered the home, she found Anthony F. sitting in a chair. His catheter had not been irrigated since he had left the hospital, although two married sons had been taught to do this before his discharge.

Neither the sons nor Catherine were willing to do it now, ostensibly because they were "afraid of contagion." In spite of explanation and reassurance by the nurse and later by the physician, this fear persisted or was used to cover some unexplained reluctance.

The family continued to keep the patient's linen and household equipment entirely separate, and his laundry was done at a different time from that of the rest of the family. The only explanation that Catherine could give was that her brothers and her aunt and her father wanted it so. Cancer, in this family, was apparently seen as a plague.

The patient was taught to irrigate the catheter himself, with Catherine willingly bringing and removing the supplies. He learned this procedure quickly. Anthony F. had always appeared to be the dominating figure in the home. His orders were quickly carried out by Catherine, who never seemed resentful but as eager to please as a preschool child.

At first, he did very well at home, although his demands were often difficult for Catherine to meet. She had always conformed to the authority of her parents. Throughout the next eleven weeks, Catherine, with the support of the visiting nurse, gave skilled nursing care to both her parents and tried to remain undisturbed by their increasingly competitive demands for her attention.

Then, as her father's physical condition worsened and his appetite, weight, and strength decreased, he became severely depressed and insisted on almost constant attention from his daughter. The visiting nurse took over more of Anthony F.'s care, but her help was never acceptable to him; he became dependent on Catherine for his entire physical care and wanted her close by him night and day.

Catherine herself had a good deal of hostility toward her parents and siblings because of the pressures on her. Yet she was bound by her training and conscience to fulfill a responsibility which she could not question.

Catherine insisted that her father remain at home to die, although alternative plans were again made available. Unable to take a stand against her family, she stated at the same time that she was unable to bear the burden of caring for him now. During the final week of illness when Anthony F. became unconscious, the visiting nurse took over more and more of his care, with Catherine assisting her. Catherine held up well throughout the terminal phase, and her father died quietly at home.

Following his death, Catherine expressed great pride in having been able "to stand it," and gradually settled into an easy and more casual relationship with her sick mother, who was now alone in the home. Her mother's needs were complex, but she was far less demanding of Catherine, and both were always able to accept a full measure of the visiting nurse's help.

After the mother's death six months later, Catherine—for the first time in her life—worked outside the home, accepting gainful employment at an unskilled job with enthusiasm. She adjusted well to it and began to make friends among her co-workers. Culture played a part, although only a part, in the behavior of both these families in a time of terminal illness. One common factor was the extent to which both families (low on the economic scale by any standards) strapped themselves financially to provide handsomely for the deceased.

Anthony F.'s family went heavily into debt to provide a most elaborate funeral for him. There were two carloads of floral wreaths leading the procession to the cemetery and this, plus elaborate expense for a handsomely-finished coffin, gave great solace to Catherine and her mother, although their own living expenses were sharply curtailed by it during the final months of the mother's life.

John T., providing new woolen blankets and a satin comforter for Mary to be buried in, proscribed their use to warm and comfort her as life ebbed in the expendable brush hogan where she died.

After her death, he asked Jean to place the red purse with all his money on Mary's body for burial. The turquoise and silver, which represented their family's wealth, was buried with her.

Charon, the boatman, was a familiar figure in ancient Greek mythology. He was the one who ferried souls across the liver Styx to the underworld of Hades. The common custom was to place coins in the mouth of the deceased so that he could be able to pay his fare across. Neither John T. nor the F. family had ever heard of this myth. Yet each, in the way of their culture, followed a similar custom, at a cost to the living.

Each family labored earnestly, or at least one member of each did, with strong approval from the others, to provide care and comfort at home before the death. Each family refused an easier way out, institutional care, although this was readily available. Each accepted medical guidance and public health nursing care throughout the whole of the terminal experience. Care by the significant helping family member was given tenderly and professional direction was sought and generally well used.

Yet in each situation, when culture directed otherwise, advice was refused. Discontinuing Mary T.'s medication and Anthony F.'s catheter irrigations represented sharp breaks with good care. No amount of teaching, explaining or requesting could overcome resistance to these unacceptable procedures. No real understanding of the underlying reasons for the resistance was ever gained.

When a public health nurse is giving care to a family whose life style is molded by a different culture, the underlying beliefs which influence behavior can often be identified, either by the giver or the recipient of care. Occasionally they cannot, or at least cannot at the time that nursing is required.

Even if the precise explanation cannot be surfaced and validated, respect for the personhood of patient and family makes it possible to continue a relationship that permits the nurse to give care effectively, while continuing the search for the cause of the behavior. That respect for personhood is among the patient's and the family's most important rights.

When, at the end of the Navajo Field Health Research and Service Program, a final report was issued: The Peoples' Health. Medicine and Anthropology in a Navajo Community (Appleton, Century Crofts, New York, 1970), it was my pleasure to find my copy autographed by the full-time staff. Almost twenty years later a revised and expanded edition of that book was published by the University of New Mexico Press (Albuquerque, 1988) and I was asked by the original authors to write the introduction to the Second Edition. It was an honor to do so.

I continued to be actively associated with the on-site staff, returning to them at intervals as a public health nursing consultant to the health visitors for several years. I saw the land and the economy change, saw improved educational programs and watched the syllabus and training manual for the health visitors' preparation become a reference for Peace Corps workers as they fanned out to developing countries abroad.

Twenty-five years after my first sight of Manyfarms, I returned to the reservation to visit the Navajo's own Community College at Tsaile. It is a college with a school of nursing headed by a Navajo dean, a dean with both doctoral preparation and wisdom in helping to keep her students rooted in their culture. I saw the school's continuing education program updating the knowledge and skills of nurses, both native and Anglo, throughout the reservation.

No segment of my nurse's career do I look back on with greater satisfaction than this association with the Navajo students as they reach out for the opportunity to serve their tribe.

Chapter 6

The Verb "To Wonder"

The verb "to wonder" has always seemed to me a special treasure of the English language. Nurse-researcher was never a title I wanted to have, perhaps because I've never been a skilled research methodologist, but rather the kind of person described so well by Bixler in the June 1942 *American Journal of Nursing:* "One who recognized nursing problems of patients and enjoyed describing and investigating these." I worked well on "the local study of limited scope which identified the larger project that needed the experienced, trained researcher."

Who said, "Chance favors the prepared mind?" I think that I have a prepared mind, in curiosity if not methodology. Another nurse and I might walk through a clinic waiting room. She could know fifty percent less than I about what was wrong with the people in the room—whose feet are hurting and swollen and what to do about it—and yet be an expert methodologist, expert in an aspect of nursing which I would never attain.

I always loved observing and putting a case history into focus or studying a "nursing incident" affecting patient care, looking at ways to measure the progress of a sick or troubled individual, perceiving common problems or conflicts requiring further definition and clarification.

Bernie Greenberg, Dean of the School of Public Health at the University of North Carolina, told me when he was chairman of the N.I.H. Nursing Studies Section that I had "an ethnographic approach" to recognizing problems for study and did well at collecting evidence which enabled the problems to be understood and wondered about by others. He counseled me to stay with to keep on perceiving relationships not yet recognized or recorded and "let others fill in the statistics." Except for a very few larger ventures, embarked on with strong help from others, that is what I have done while giving or teaching direct patient care.

I would not want to be a full-time researcher. I've never thought of myself as any kind of scholar. I like to do things for people. In fact, for the first half of my life I was convinced that I never wanted-ed to teach at all; I just wanted to "do." Then I got into teaching accidentally and found that I liked it. In my kind of teaching, anyhow, I'd still be doing.

I never especially wanted to learn statistics. Of course, I did learn it, after all. But I was curious. I'd see situations in patient care and I'd begin to do little mini-projects to find a better solution.

Let's say I was doing public health nursing and I found it was very difficult to get private physicians to change their orders, even though it was perfectly obvious from the observations I made and from the memos I sent to the doctors that something else was indicated.

So my way of handling my own frustrations when they would send back new orders that simply said, "Continue as before," was to say "I'll take the next twenty situations in which I've got good evidence that orders ought to be changed and I'll just assign numbers to them from the table of random numbers." (O.K., so I used a little bit of statistical knowledge.) "And in the ones that end with an even number, I'll do exactly what I did before, send a very good memo to the doctor, spelling out what I thought should be changed. In the other group, the odd numbers, I'll make a personal phone call to the doctor, outlining my perceptions of the patient's needs, and ask him for his judgment." I was asking the doctor to get the patient into better focus, to *help me with his thinking* and not just with his signature. And that was always the approach that worked.

These mini-projects that I became involved with identified a problem and described its occurrence in multiple settings or set up simple variables, like the telephone study, that might lead to a solution. They brought surprises to light or led to bigger investigations later. I had never even heard the term *nursing research* when I did the very first of these.

1948. "Nursing Care Can Be Measured"

Faced with a tough problem on night duty about which I had a hunch and some natural variables, I set up three data-collection columns on the inside cover of the narcotic book, collected evidence for a month and documented the probable validity of the hunch.

The problem, as I saw it, was the overuse of sedatives on an Army hospital ward at bedtime. I believed that, with an extra hour of attention—back rubs, refilled water pitchers, a doctor's visit— we could reduce the need for sedation. Friendliness, and the pleasanter, more relaxed atmosphere, resulted in the use of 33 to 45 percent less narcotics and sedatives being administered.

A year later, discharged from the Army, I had a part-time job at the *Journal of Nursing* while attending graduate school. A golden bonus of this work was having frequent lunches with Mary Roberts, then the Journal's editor. One day she spoke to me about the need for nursing to measure patient care. That evening I hunted up the notes from my sedatives experiment and the next day I gave them to her. I shall always remember the excitement in her voice when she said, "Miss Schwartz, you've measured patient care!" Published in five paragraphs on two-thirds of a page, that mini-study was replicated widely.

Other similar mini-studies followed, although they varied considerably in content.

1953. "Health Promotional Literature for Clinic Patients"

Here, the question was why some health promotional literature seemed to be disappearing from a particular clinic. Why were elderly, diabetic patients removing pamphlets about child growth and development and about normal nutrition at an unprecedented rate? Who was using this and to what purpose? We found that we had been unaware of the fine diagnostic tool we already had at our disposal.

To learn more about this phenomenon, we limited the number of pamphlets and labeled them: "If you think a personal copy will help you, talk with the nurse about obtaining one." The answer was staring us in the face. People had been taking our literature home to read and help with health problems there. Patients don't simply leave family concerns at the clinic door when they come for personal health treatment.

Their responses resulted in "literature-motivated" patient con-ferences—brief, productive interchanges between patient and nurse. New health problems the staff was unaware of came to light, as well as an increased awareness by staff of the nature of patients' interests and concerns about matters of health.

When the study was finished, I realized that I had no idea how to write it up how to structure the report. I wrote the paragraphs that were examples, described stories about the patients. A statis-tician helped me with the tables. But what about the conclusion and summary? Dr. George Reader, professor of medicine at Cornell (now professor of public health) invited me to his office one Saturday morning. I spent hours writing and he spent hours criticizing.

I've never had any trouble writing the summary and conclusion of an article since then. So when I'm asked, did I have training as a researcher, the answer is, yes I had training, but informal train-ing. It was on the spot. That was really my first planned study. It subsequently was published in the *American Journal of Public Health,* a difficult journal to get into. But it was unusual and sim-ple and obvious enough so that it was picked up right away. And because that journal has a tremendous international outreach, there came almost immediately requests for reprints from Russia, Australia, the Middle East and India, from fairly top people in out-lying places.

As I go over it now, it's still a small, good paper and I'm proud of it.

1958. "Uncooperative Patients?"

An attempt to categorize nonconformists in a busy clinic brought about a new definition of "difficult" patients. The enemy, it seemed, turned out to be us. This was really a project of my undergraduate students. Students came to me with a problem: "How come you say there's no such thing as an uncooperative patient and yet everybody around here says that so-and-so is uncooperative?" Well, students usually ask good questions. And when they complain about faculty, it's usually worth thinking about what the faculty is doing.

So I said, "I don't really know why we call patients uncooperative; why if the patient does this, he's uncooperative, but if he does that, he's not uncooperative. Nothing that I could give you as an explanation makes any sense, not only to you but to me. So why don't we try to figure out together what the answer is?"

What we needed to do first was to find out who was considered uncooperative by the staff. One person, or perhaps one discipline, says that somebody is being uncooperative. Maybe it's the professional who does the calling who really is uncooperative, not the patient. We needed to identify who is considered an uncooperative patient in this clinic by *all* the different professionals. That would not tell us that he's really uncooperative, only that he's a patient who an awful lot of people believe is uncooperative.

Now, we wouldn't just be able to go around and say, "Who do you think is an uncooperative patient?" Because everybody knows that it's considered professionally irresponsible to call anybody uncooperative. We have to think up a way of asking them that isn't going to put any staff member on the spot. They're going to have to help identify something without feeling that we are making them vulnerable.

The students worked on it and they figured out the way to do it was to say, "A patient in this clinic is called uncooperative. Who do you think that might be?" You are not asking the worker to call him uncooperative. **You** are calling him uncooperative. **You** are saying, whom do you think of?

And so they got a list of fifty patients every discipline working in the clinic considered uncooperative, fifty patients who seemed not willing even to come in through the door. Apparently they flew in on broomsticks. They had the ability to get everybody's hackles up.

"Now let's get their charts and see what the common denominators are. What disease, diagnosis, or personal characteristics did they have in common?"

So we worked over the fifty charts. We couldn't find anything. They had nothing in common that we could identify. If there were fifty different types of patients in that clinic, they were the fifty different types. They went from our youngest to our oldest, equal proportions of men and women, every medical diagnosis known in the clinic. Then we were at our wit's end when we found that there were people who were much more hostile than these fifty but who were not considered uncooperative.

And then it began to turn out that some of the staff thought our fifty really were unappreciative patients. "Oh, so we want people to be grateful to us?" These people weren't. They didn't appreciate how much we were doing for them. O.K. Maybe we had something there. Each staff member says it differently but it amounts to the same thing, "He makes me feel ineffective."

Patients who get better do a great service to the nurses and doctors who are responsible for their care. But it's not exactly that. These patients are not failing to get better. Or, if some of them are failing, so too are other patients who are not being labeled uncooperative. So what do these patients do besides not getting better? "They make me feel ineffective."

And this is the best definition I've ever found for an uncooperative patient. The staff person says, "I'm trying as hard as I can.

But I not only fail to succeed, I feel myself a failure for failing to succeed." When a patient doesn't get better, in effect, it's a personal insult to the helping person. So he responds with anger and depression. And the anger breaks whatever good relationship may have existed and makes the patient less inclined to try and the caretaker less satisfied with the care he or she is able to provide. At that point, there is something wrong with what is being done for the patient, whereas initially there probably wasn't.

1962. "The Elderly Ambulatory Patient"

By 1962 I had obtained my first grant and gained released time for a longer study. I was trying to find out how elderly patients who were chronically ill with several afflictions were managing to live at home. This was actually several separate studies of various activities of daily living, all the data for which we gathered simultaneously so that it could be examined subject by subject: diet, medication habits, ambulation and travel, leisure time activities and so on. The information was coded so that one could look at each part of a separate mini-study but could also call up an individual profile of every participating respondent to improve that patient's care.

In all the previous small projects, I had been the only investigator. This one required three people: an anthropologist, who was a superb statistician; a social worker; and myself as a public health nurse. We were equals in the study, although I was principal investigator; I wrote the grant. We hired graduate nurses and two student nurses—partly to give them work-study opportunities, but also to help me in teaching them.

Each study was published separately and then the total picture was combined into a book, *The Elderly Ambulatory Patient: Nursing and Psychosocial Needs.* (Schwartz, Doris, Barbara Henley, and

Leonard Zeitz. New York: Macmillan, 1964.) We used a very careful sampling of 220 patients who represented 2,200 who were coming into the clinic and met the necessary criteria.

I talked to each of the 220 (or as many as I could find who hadn't moved or died in the meantime) and the social worker on the study talked to them, separately. It seemed as though our people were coping primarily in one of four ways.

This was not something that we had been looking for; it turned up as a result. When we coded all the protocols and ran them through the computer, they simply fell into four profiles.

1. The sick person who was well cared for by an apparently adequate spouse.

2. The patient who no longer could maintain independence in living and had moved in to live with a married child.

3. The old person without family ties who lived in a rooming house.

4. The husband and wife who were both sick and mutually dependent.

Extensive case histories illustrated the reports of this study, offering anecdotal material as well as analysis of the histories.

The findings from this investigation were mixed. On the one hand, it was found that the elderly were clearly a subject for further nursing and interdisciplinary research, that the attempt to categorize this group in gerontological terms had real validity. (This subject had been controversial at the time the proposal had been submitted.) The data indicated that much further research and action was needed to design supportive accommodations or to improve living facilities for the frail elderly population. The book

also played a useful part in stimulating nurses to define for themselves a role as researchers as well as caregivers.

Ironically, it gave me a reputation that was to prove somewhat
embarrassing, of being perceived more as an academician than the
clinical teacher that I tried so hard to be.

Now that a decent interval of almost thirty years has passed, I
can look back on this work and justify many of the concerns
included in it by current developments that grew out of the major
topic.

For example, from the small focus on medication-taking behavior of patients, previous studies of which had tended to concentrate on a single drug, a vast literature has grown on error-making
and the reasons for such. Such reasons cover the behavior of the
prescriber and instructor (the individual who gives directions to
the patient) as well as the behavior of the "non-conformist" patient
or the elderly confused patient with several medications to take.

The report of the comprehensive interrelated study has been
cited as "a pioneer investigation" in the journals of other professions: medicine, pharmacy, sociology, social work. While always
recognized as a "beginning study," whose findings showed the
need for more detailed data and a wider spectrum of respondents,
it now can be considered as one of the early studies to look at nursing needs of patients as indicators of culture, life style, and coping
ability.

Although not the intent of the study, it documented strengths,
weaknesses and—above all—differences in the way physicians,
nurses and social workers sought information from patients and
what they did with such information when it became available.

1986. "Alternatives to Restraints"

Today, I'm interested in what I consider the overuse of
restraints on confused elderly people. There had been very little

research done here. Tying someone into a wheelchair or a bed, not letting him have full control of himself, may be essential temporarily, for some dangerous situations in order to keep a confused person from hurting himself or someone else.

I'm not talking about someone who is comatose and unable to control his own body motions and who would slide out of a chair, but rather someone who is restrained against his or her will, to keep him from wandering off. There is a growing amount of this, in part because there are growing numbers of older people who are in hospitals and nursing homes and partly because of the complex surgical procedures now undertaken.

This means that many chronically ill patients who are confused or mentally ill, or brain-failed for whatever reason, are often being cared for by fewer or less well-prepared staff. Therefore it is easier to keep these patients strapped into chairs. There will be fewer people walking around with whom one must become involved.

I would like to see some real research conducted in nursing homes and the kind of hospital units that tend to have older patients. (In a ward of persons with fractured hips, almost everyone is likely to be elderly.) I would suggest having a T.V. monitor in such a place. Of course, since this is an invasion of privacy, permission would have to be secured.

What one gets usually is only the staff's story of why the patient is being restrained. "We restrain him for his own safety," is the usual explanation. Only by having an observer (in person or through the television monitor) is it possible to know what interaction took place between the restrained and the restrainer, and what alternatives were tried, if any.

What seems to label a patient "uncooperative" is that he or she fails to do the will of a professional person. The professional responds in kind and is ashamed of it. Then the patient is treated as uncooperative. I believe this may be the cause of restraint abuse in many situations, particularly if it is a confused elderly patient.

The investigation of effective nursing alternatives to restraints is only just beginning, and I am on the sidelines cheering on those who presently are seeking solutions. Happily, several of my nursing colleagues at the University of Pennsylvania (notably Neville Strumpf and Lois Evans) are as eager to explore alternatives to restraints as am I. Since they are younger, with more time ahead of them than I, and are joined by many others across the country (both professionals and advocacy groups), I look forward to vast improvement in reducing restraints over the next decade.

For most of my years at Cornell-New York Hospital, it was my privilege to work alongside a wonderful nurse-colleague, Mamie Wong. She had been educated at the Peking Union Medical College's School of Nursing in the 1930s. Many of the mini-studies during the 1950s and 1960s grew out of observations first made by Mamie, who tugged at me to wonder about what occurred in the clinic on a daily basis. She became my mentor and my conscience through an amusing kind of interaction.

Mamie always was a superb patient advocate and for some years (as I remember it now) she would resign regularly every Friday afternoon. As the clinic emptied and she came to say goodnight, she would repeat a refrain which I grew to know very well:

"Doris, I cannot continue to work in this clinic. We are not meeting the nursing needs of the patients well enough. My letter of resignation is on your desk."

"Mamie, what troubles you at this time to the point of sending your letter of resignation?"

"Doris, this is a very busy clinic. There are many patients with problems, with which referrals or our own teaching could be of help. With present staffing we have only two or three minutes of face-to-face contact with each person to get to know them. What do we do with that small piece of time? We seal the patient's mouth closed with a thermometer."

"Mamie, suppose instead of my acting on your letter of resignation tonight, you keep it until Monday and then tell us Monday morning how we should go about increasing our talking and listening time with patients."

"I will suggest a way for you on Monday."

And Mamie always did, because her mind truly put into practice the meaning of the phrase "all things considered." Like Sinclair Lewis's character Dr. Martin Arrowsmith, she "had one gift: a curiosity whereby (s)he saw nothing as ordinary." Mamie Wong is an extraordinary nurse who helped me to continue to wonder about everything we were doing in those exciting years of nursing progress. I thank her for her inspiration.

Chapter 7

The World Health Organization's "Expert Committee on Nursing"

In the Spring of 1966 I was invited to become a member of the fourth Expert Committee on Nursing called by the World Health Organization (W.H.O.). Expert Committees are convened to give advice to the W.H.O. on scientific and technical matters. Members of the expert groups serve without remuneration, in their personal capacity, and not as representatives of their governments or other bodies.

I am not quite sure what led to this invitation; around this time I had been doing a good deal of writing in the literature and perhaps that is why I was contacted. At any rate I was enormously pleased. There was a stop on my way to Geneva, in Edinburgh, Scotland. It was customary at the time for universities, even nations, to ask W.H.O. for help in health problems or in teaching and for committee members to stop off and do double duty as consultants on the way to the W.H.O. meeting.

I was sent to the University of Edinburgh to offer several classes to a group of W.H.O.-sponsored international nurses studying
there and to discuss with them and the School of Nursing faculty
recent U.S. nursing research. The stopover made my European
leave even more fascinating and worthwhile.

As all Expert Committees do, ours completed a collective report
published in the W.H.O. Technical Report Series. These reports do
not necessarily represent the views of the organization, but they
are taken into serious consideration for the development of future
programs.

During the seventies I was asked by W.H.O. to serve on the first
Expert Committee on Geriatric Care, which had become a specialty of mine by then.

April 24, 1966. At J.F. Kennedy Airport, I got aboard one of
those B.O.A.C. Rolls Royce 707s. We took off on schedule at 8 p.m.,
passed over Nantucket in due course, and about two hours out (on
a six-hour flight to London) the plane began to feel not quite the
way it usually does.

Shortly thereafter, the captain announced that, to his regret, we
would have to dump 10,000 gallons of fuel into the Atlantic and go
back; the plane's hydraulic controls were not functioning correctly
and he couldn't identify the trouble.

The B.O.A.C. people were superb; they'd have made fine recovery room personnel in their cool, friendly, concerned handling of
everyone and everything. Back at Kennedy Airport, by the time it
became clear that the plane couldn't fly that night, it was 3 a.m.,
with 140 people to find hotel rooms for and get transferred to other
airlines as quickly as possible.

The next day I took off on T.W.A., arriving in London at midnight (Wednesday) and just missing the last flight to Edinburgh.

My class was scheduled for Thursday at 9:30 a.m. at Edinburgh University. I spent the rest of the night in London Airport and went up on the 8 a.m. shuttle. A cheerful Scots driver who was ready to cope with anything pulled me up in front of the International School of Nursing on the university campus, bags and all, with me looking a trifle haggard, at 9:27 a.m. As he said, "A full three minutes to spare, lassie."

The Internationals are a group of about thirty nurses being prepared for senior positions in their home countries in nursing education or nursing service. W.H.O. sponsors this certificate program for senior personnel of extraordinary promise (advanced supervision or advanced education) so that they can get cracking at setting up degree programs in nursing for young people who today are getting the backgrounds needed for university matriculation.

My two days there consisted of two formal lectures, which were really quite informal, and then hourly conferences, by appointment, with these students from the international group. I discussed patient-care research ideas they had for their home countries, or talked with faculty doing research, who were primarily hungry to know pertinent reference material from ongoing U.S. studies.

As a matter of fact, all the faculty seem deep in nursing research. Miss Elsie Stephenson, director of the nursing school, was nurse investigator of two of that country's great interdisciplinary family health studies: "1,000 Families in Newcastle on Tyne" (Spence, Walden *et al.*), and "The Health of the Elderly in Edinburgh" (Williams). Certain hours of the week are released for faculty research, as well as certain summer time.

Their student body is only about half of ours in number, however, and they in no way are yet able to control the undergraduate student's clinical practice. Great classroom teaching, but the students are pretty much thrown to the wolves on the wards and in the public health nursing agencies. And the ward sisters (head nurses) of the Royal Infirmary at Edinburgh seem to have not changed much since Lister's time.

One or two of the sisters still live on the wards, I am told, sleeping in the sisters' room and being awakened daily by the junior (student) night nurse, with a steaming pot of tea.

"Good morning, Sister, it's six o'clock. May I give you the night report?"

A couple of recent graduates assured me that some of those veteran sisters could open one eye, peer through the teapot's steam, and within forty seconds get an accurate account of every misdeed of the nighttime staff, so comprehensive was their knowledge of all the potential errors, oversights and blunders a student nurse could make. In any event, the place still looks as it did when William Ernest Henley wrote the wonderful collection of poems called "In Hospital" there in 1875, although some of the most exciting breakthroughs in medicine are coming from that place today.

The whole Edinburgh campus is enormously lively. I stayed at the staff house (faculty club), which has only a few guest rooms but is the center of eating, drinking, arguing, debating, pool playing, and dart throwing for hundreds of university staff: old and young. The building buzzed and hummed from crack of dawn till midnight with scholars and would-be ones.

Scottish universities are a clan unto themselves; membership in any university student organization or faculty club gives one reciprocal rights to use the counterpart at every other Scottish university. So there's a great deal of informal interchanging.

Both evenings, groups of faculty had very informal dinners in someone's flat. If Edinburgh has had new buildings put up in the last eighty years I didn't see any of them; only elegant old grey sandstone blocks of five story flats.

The people are not unlike the Navajo. They won't be swayed by anything modern unless convinced that it's better than what they've got. Which means that Scotland adopted plumbing, electricity, and wonderful hot towel racks in the lofty bathrooms very early, and then, by cracky, not a thing new has been added for forty years. At least not in the buildings of the colleagues who took me into their homes.

April 28. A pleasant one-hour flight brought me to Switzerland, and a room at the appointed hotel. It is really a *pension* rather than a hotel, serving breakfast only, but it is quiet and homelike, looks out on a lovely backyard garden, and is within walking distance of the Palais des Nations.

The Palais is an incredibly beautiful setting. The lovely buildings of the palace are in a large park of flowering trees on the edge of Geneva's Lake Leman. The snow-capped mountains ring the city, and on a clear day we can see Mont Blanc from the conference room window.

This building was built for the League of Nations and many of the major peace conferences of the world have been held here. The carpet in the meeting room is worn down to the warp, and one sits in the session listening to the phenomena of simultaneous translation of the speakers' comments on the left and right, from French into English, and it is impossible not to wonder whose feet have scuffed the carpet—and over what international issues?

One watches the intelligent faces of the translators in the booths at the end of the room and marvels at their skill in transmitting just the right shade of your fellow committee-woman's meaning. Then you wonder what great events they've translated, in this self-same room, for others who sat at this table.

You talk with them about this whole astonishing process of simultaneous translation at the coffee break, and they share with you the excitement of translating for the Big Four meeting, and tell you of instances when the whole fabric of a touchy conference hinged on or was hindered by the fortunate or unfortunate translation of a single idiom.

Happily for them—and us—there is little pressure for finding the right choice of words at this particular committee meeting; everyone is extraordinarily clear in expressing herself (or himself). But it is a most extraordinary feeling to put on an earphone and or hear what you are saying in English rendered into careful French even while you are literally in mid-sentence. I've listened to similar translation at the United Nations, of course, but never thought that I'd participate in such a session.

Our chairman is a lawyer and dean of a Philippine school of nursing. Vice chairman is the nurse from the Ministry of Health of Poland. *Rapporteur* (recorder) is the nurse from the Ministry of Health of England. The ranking nurse from W.H.O. (a Canadian) is with them at the head of the table.

Around the table are fourteen nurses and three doctors representing Mexico, Ghana, Finland, Belgium, Iran, Greece, U.S.A., France, Sweden, Brazil, India, Canada, etc. In the center of the table is the electronic equipment for translation—much the same sort of wiring required in a coronary care unit.

The task of this committee is to issue a report, by the end of next week, that will spell out guidelines for improving the quality of nursing care, while maintaining the quantity of care, all around the world. I think all of us feel the need for a little touch of magic. The French word for session is *séance* and a seance is what the committee, indeed, would wish for each time it meets.

You may wonder what other *séances* are being held here simultaneously? The big bulletin board in the lobby which lists the *séances* publique and *séances privat* each morning, today read:

Expert Committee on Lead and Zinc Poisoning

Expert Committee on Rheumatic Fever

Expert Committee on Nursing

European Economic Community

Committee on the Peaceful Uses of Outer Space

Committee on U.N. Finances

Scientific and Technical Sub Committee

In our own session when one speaks of developing countries' problems, one always says carefully, "I refer to the problems of countries in the process of technological development." Early on, the nurse from Ghana and the nurse from Iran found it necessary "to remind the representatives of the nations from the so-called European and American cultures that Iran and Ghana had thousands of years of history recorded in art and literature and lore transmitted in epic poetry, and they would prefer not to be considered developing countries in comparison to some whose technological development perhaps exceeded their development in the humanities."

The point was well taken and we all are more careful to say what we mean, which is really a categorization of countries developing technologically, countries with a great deal of technological know-how, and countries whose technology is now moving swiftly into automation.

There is another way of putting it. I notice that the African representatives here (the young woman from our committee, a physician from Nigeria on the Expert Committee on Rheumatic Fever and the deputy Minister of Health from Tanzania) always use the terms "the young countries and the older ones," although reference to technology, which is only beginning in a young country, is quite acceptable.

Exceptions are frequently taken to a particular word because its meaning is very different in the represented countries. The rewording is always done with great care to preserve the meaning, to clarify the concept, and to scale whatever obstacle presented itself. The definition of nurse was one such example. So, too, was the need to identify the most responsibly prepared nurses in each country while recognizing that the level of preparation varied from country to country in a manner difficult to comprehend.

Interesting items: In Cambodia, all student nurses are men; top priority is the recruitment of women into nursing. In Korea there are no jobs for graduate nurses. Students provide all the services for the hospitals and public health nursing units. No one wants to pay money for the graduate product when the student can be exploited for board and room and training.

Training, incidentally, is a concept over which we've spent a lot of time and I am convinced that it was discarded too rapidly by the U.S. as a dirty word. Both education and training appear to have a proper place in the learning of a discipline which is professional, but, after all, if someone in this conference room were to suffer a cardiac arrest, who would he or she rather be sitting next to—a person who could give a scholarly paper on the cardiopulmonary system or someone so well-trained in cardiopulmonary resuscitation that the practice of it was almost automatic?

April 29. The sessions I've attended are warmly informal in the lively give-and-take but the atmosphere is one of great dignity. One addresses the Chair, "Madam Chairman, I would like to say"…Or, if speaking in French, "Madame La Presidente—." And one always closes a comment with "Thank you, Madam Chairman" or "*Merci*, Madame La Presidente."

At the start of each session we are reminded that within the W.H.O. we do not represent any single country but speak for ourselves, with concern for the health problems of the world. The experience which each of us brings, however, from intimate knowledge of the conditions of the country from which she comes is something that all present will benefit from.

One often presents facts by saying, "In my country, such and such occurs," but it is clear that we are progressively thinking more in terms of the "technologically developing," "technologically developed" and "technologically moving toward automation" with each *séance*. Out of session—at meals or over drinks—one argues politics of one's own or any other country with fervor.

I have felt the need to get to the library and take out (for bedtime reading) David Coyle's *The American Political System and How It Works*, which, it appears, has been recently translated into the Indonesian, Bengali, Marathi, Gujarati, Urdu, Tamil, Hindi, Malayalam Arabic, Greek, French, Spanish, Chinese and Japanese languages. It ill behooves an English-speaking American citizen abroad to be without an explanation of the meaning of some paragraph of this comment on "democracy at work," while in the Palais cafeteria. I had known of the book but had never read it, and for the life of me, I hadn't known of the existence of some of the languages it has been translated into. Happily, I can now discuss the English language version, and very useful it seems to be.

My primary paper, "Quality of Nursing Care" has now been presented and discussed. I have one more hurdle: being first discussant on the topic, "Nursing Research in Patient Care," and then possibly a sub-committee assignment for drafting a portion of the report for Monday. Sunday we are all taking a holiday.

May 2. The weather has become progressively better, with the last few days showing spring at its best. Within the city there are beds and boxes and elaborate plantings of tulips everywhere, while in the country whole mountainsides and fields are ablaze with brilliant field-flowers of gold and bright blue.

Two great categories of problems stand out in every hour of meeting time: the problem of language and differences of culture which each language represents, and the problem of poverty throughout most of the world. Whatever the point of discussion, and whatever aspect of nursing we are emphasizing, someone is sure to bring the talk down to the basic fact that truly scientific practice is unrealistic when most of the babies a nurse sees in her part of the world are in advanced stages of starvation.

"Individualizing nutrition teaching within the framework of the family's preferences" has no meaning at all to a family in Calcutta whose total intake for the day is one handful of boiled rice apiece bought out-of-doors from an almost equally poor vendor who has set up his caldron over a fire on a busy corner and boiled up a huge pot. People approach him with two coppers (2/100s of one rupee), for which he scoops rice from the pot with his bare hands and puts it into the bare hands of the buyer, while passers-by without two coppers stand around and dive like seagulls to pick up the individual rice grains that have spilled during this transaction.

One of our committee has recently been to Mecca during the annual Arab pilgrimage. The pilgrimage, of course, attracts literally hundreds of thousands of Moslems from all over, and she reported evidence of significant malnutrition in that population.

But again, the real problem in every clinic, outweighing every other diagnostic and therapeutic consideration, is enough food to keep a population alive long enough to be nursed. Even control of smallpox becomes insignificant by comparison. One of our group was told by a local health official, "In all of India last year we had 250,000 cases of smallpox, only some of whom actually died. Why are you worried by this? Many times this many are dying of starvation, literally dying of it, or dying of malnutrition. Why don't you use the priorities you talk about?"

In this setting, the problems of talking about worldwide nursing (patient care, nursing systems, the administration of nursing service, and nursing research) sometime lose perspective to the point that in the lunch hour one walks past the room where the disarmament conferences have been in continuous session for four years or more and the whole bleak picture of human stupidity momentarily takes precedence over everything else. Then one gets it into focus again and returns to the problem of moving on with planning for one small segment of the human race, that segment who wish to nurse more than to destroy.

You discover, as the discussion continues, that in some of the countries of the world the whole year's quota of student nurses are selected as a batch, without any consideration of where each will go to school and with no recognition of individual differences in either students or schools. In fact, the term used to describe the annual intake is "a parcel." It becomes difficult in teaching a parcel to personalize—or repersonalize—the patient.

That bane of our own students' vocabulary, "preparation for leadership" turns up. Here we strike real fire. The translators nod to one another in the booths. The problem is a new one to the committee members but the translators have met it many times before in conferences of all types.

"What is this leadership quality you Americans constantly talk about? It has ruined the foreign student fellowships for many of us. There is no translation for this concept in other languages! The qualities you call leadership are not called leadership in my country. They are called guidance or management qualities. Leadership is the innate quality of being able to lead." And again, the word "professional." We are told, "Professional is American jargon. There is nothing wrong with these words: professional and leadership, in English, only because your sociologists have attached them to values which you comprehend. But in my language (Finnish, Iranian, Portuguese) they have no translation."

(I think then of a day—out in Arizona—when Ken Denison, our Navajo consultant, sat with me in the car outside a hogan and explained why the thought of an adult Navajo leading any other adult Navajo was demeaning. Yet both Ken and our committee member accepted the importance of good practitioners of nursing as role models. In fact, the lack of a sufficient number of practitioners who are good role models disturbed them both.)

All over the world one problem of nursing is agreed on: that nursing schools have been operated in total isolation from organized educational institutions. A major effort of this committee will be to reverse this trend in its recommendations.

Nevertheless, the system of any country's education, and the primary and secondary school educational opportunities for women, will have to determine what kind of an organized educational institution a school of nursing might fit into.

Two other problems are worldwide. One can be stated, "Personnel are enticed for a particular technical function which is ephemeral, rather than being recruited into a nursing system which meets the broad needs of a people." The other problem on which both sophisticated and unsophisticated educational programs were in agreement was a sad one: "Teaching presents the easiest way out of actual patient care. How can we insure that those who teach know how to care for patients?"

A third point isn't exactly a problem but in some ways it is. From the bottom of a committeeman or committeewoman's heart from time to time comes the wish, impossible to attain, "I wish we could stand still for one year ... if change only didn't come so fast." It is this incredible narrowing of the span of time available for decision making which is the least common denominator of every fraction. This makes all countries become concerned with training their students (and teachers) for uncertainty, for the setting of priorities in a constantly changing world.

There have been several delightfully humorous moments. At one point almost every nation felt called upon to list the qualities of an ideal nurse. I don't quite know how this got started. It was certainly no one's intention to compile such a laundry list but someone mentioned the characteristics needed by the best-prepared persons in nursing.

Someone else expanded on them, and it was late in the day and everyone was tired and before we knew it, there was the list of girl-scout attributes being expanded at a great pace. This went on for several minutes until finally an elderly doctor from Afghanistan (who had come in as a spectator) asked and received permission to address the chair. "Surely, Madam Chairman, these nurses whom you speak about must be daughters of God."

We seem to mention the things that get in the way of smooth committee work more often than the scads of things we're all agreed upon. That is because such details impede the progress of this constant drive to cover the agenda and get the report into final form. By W.H.O. regulations, a technical committee's report must be in final draft and signed by the participants before adjournment.

We completed our first draft Saturday morning and discussed it with a snowstorm of suggestions for change. A subcommittee worked on the revisions Sunday, while the rest of us took off on the Chillon excursion. This morning we took the second draft apart but it's most interesting to see the progress being made toward agreement. Now the discussion is only rarely a disagreement, usually a rewording of or clarifying a point "to make it more useful in countries like mine."

Tomorrow is the opening of the World Health Assembly, which is about as colorful as the start of the U.N. Assembly in New York. We will recess for the morning to attend the opening ceremony. Later in the week I will have three days of touring: one-day trips into the Swiss and Italian Alps, returning each night to Geneva, to simplify packing and moving in this brief stretch of time.

I have spent most of my leisure in the close company of three companions, not to the exclusion of the others but because we all like walking, we have been together coming and going, and we tend to have our meals together. One is the young Moslem nurse from Iran, one the stately and striking woman from Ghana, and the other the nurse from the Polish government's Ministry of Health. Politics, everyday life in these countries, community organization and recipes from the four countries' kitchens make extremely interesting table conversation.

May 11. Yesterday I returned home with the final draft of our committee's report and the preliminary papers to share with the Cornell colleagues who were holding down the fort during my absence, proving that I was, after all, dispensable. Now I return to the midterms and term papers, still ungraded, of my very patient students.

From World Health to Public Health, as it is taught in one class in one nursing school in one city in America.

Chapter 8

The Nurse as Primary Practitioner

"A chief aim of the Comprehensive Care and Teaching Program is the development of a comprehensive, fully adequate, continuing type of medical care, which may be copied on an economic and feasible basis and which might furnish the model for excellent medical care for all of the people."

David Barr, M.D.
Professor of Medicine
Cornell Medical College

These words, written in 1951 at the start of the Cornell Medical College's Comprehensive Care and Teaching Program, became the legend of the program. It was framed and hung on the wall of the waiting room in the General Medical Clinic.

I had only one reservation about this attractive aim. I should have liked it to substitute "health care" for "medical care." When I started to work in the program as a staff nurse in the General Medical Clinic I hoped to introduce the principles and practice of public health nursing into the clinic's daily routine.

George Reader, professor of medicine and director of the Comprehensive Care and Teaching Program, was welcoming but doubtful. He was unable to discern a specific role for public health nursing practice in this new interdisciplinary teaching program for senior medical students. Kathleen Newton, author of the nation's first geriatric nursing textbook and director of out-patient nursing, told me to keep a low profile but to take advantage of every chance to introduce public health concepts to the patients and students.

"Do it," Kay said, "but don't talk about it yet. Let them discover what you are doing."

The goal was to identify a wider spectrum of needs of patients and families and to help medical students recognize and meet them. Neither Kay nor I realized that we were on the edge of what was to become a new pattern of medicine: family practice. What nurses did as a matter of course would in time be recognized and valued by the medical students.

And so, in those early years in the Comprehensive Care and Teaching Program, I anticipated the later preparation of family nurse practitioners, and the orientation of medical students in the program presaged the coming emphasis on their discipline's family practice.

In one of his first papers dealing with the program, Professor Reader was to comment that:

> "raising the nurse and social worker to full partnership
> with the physician in directing patient management has

produced a significant alteration in medical care and teaching. The constant seeking of the nurse to find and fulfill patients' needs and the nondirective approach of the social worker have come as a revelation to the physician, who is ordinarily blinded to total patient needs by his desire to diagnose a disease entity and overpowered by his urge to treat the patient actively." ("Organization and Development of a Comprehensive Care Program." *American Journal of Public Health,* Vol. 44, No. 6, June 1954.)

During the final decade of my twenty-nine-year span at Cornell (1951-80) we started and carried to completion one of the first government-funded family nurse practitioner programs—known as Primex—and followed it with one of the first educational programs for the preparation of geriatric nurse practitioners.

January 1971. Primex was conceptualized to prepare nurses in the delivery of primary health care. To me, primary care is simply the first point of professional contact, whenever the need for help is recognized. This care might be given by a physician, as had been done by general practitioners for many years.

It could be, and was, given to certain populations by the staff nurses of our most imaginative public health nursing agencies, under Visiting Nurse or Health Department auspices, although generally they had been academically prepared to give only certain segments of it.

Bill Mauldin's great cartoons of the mud-beleaguered infantrymen of World War II show that it had been given, too, by para-professionals long before Mr. Webster and his successors had entered the phrase "primary care" in the dictionary. The front-line medical corpsman who recognized that "crisis care" alone was not enough to keep any army moving was, in a very real sense, a primary practitioner at work.

I am thinking about a range of health services, at varying levels of depth, offered close to where the recipient is. These would include concem for primary and secondary prevention, case finding, accurate assessment, sound treatment of those health problems which the practitioner is competent to treat, fast and able referral of problems beyond the practitioner's competency, and a deep concem for understanding the system in which the patient lives and works: his culture, the monitoring required to maintain his health, and the minutiae of detail required in rehabilitation measures which are needed to return him to his everyday life and keep him there productively.

This involves recognition of a patient's needs, interaction of the patient with his health problems in his life setting, and an awareness of the altemative approaches to coping and of what help other health professionals and agencies are able to give. Nurses were already bringing such skills to health-care settings, without additional preparation. With further preparation the nurse's role could expand in terms of case finding, the defining and management of health problems, as well as in health education and planning.

In the past, it generally took two persons, peripherally related and with little overlap (a physician and a public health nurse) to deliver all the services required by many families in their natural setting. Other families—by the thousands—required this spread of services but did not have it simply because the human resources were not available. It seemed necessary to meld the two parent-disciplines into a single agent of care. This frees highly prepared specialists and institutions for situations where their know-how and resources can make a significant difference. The hypothesis is that melding these parent-disciplines in a nurse who chooses the primary role can be superior for some clients to even the best traditional community health nursing or medical practice.

"The candidate for Primex Programs will be a registered nurse already working in community health nursing agencies such as V.N.A.s, Health Departments, organized home-care programs, day centers for older citizens, clinics, nursing homes, and hospitals with unusually large populations of chronically-ill older patients, such as Veterans Administration hospitals."

At the start we developed a conceptual framework for viewing the nurse practitioner's role. This includes an understanding of how to maintain a steady state in the complex human organism, which involves some gross anatomy, basic physiology, and system physiology. Then came knowledge and skill in assessing the health status of an individual: didactic and practice sessions in history taking, performance of a complete physical examination, the use of problem lists, and plans for therapy and approach.

Fall, 1971. Primex at Cornell was a year-long continuing education program. The one-year curriculum consisted of an intensive four-and-one-half month didactic semester, including closely supervised clinical practice in an ambulatory-care setting, followed by a seven-and-one-half month internship in the nurse's community agency, working in close collaboration with medical and nursing preceptors. An additional 120 contact hours of classroom content were built into the internship period. The initial idea for a Primex Program at Cornell was Dean Eleanore Lambertsen's. The first outline for the curriculum was planned jointly by Dean Lambertsen, Eva Reese, Director of the Visiting Nurse Service of New York, and myself.

Clinical experience was offered in the general medical clinic and in a satellite clinic of the hospital, held at a community center within two large public-housing projects where there was an exceptionally high occupancy rate of elderly tenants. These medical clinics served four main categories of patients:

1. The person with many complaints and multiple disorders—often long-standing chronic illnesses in good, fair or poor control.

2. The person with a true diagnostic problem who is sometimes best served by a specialty clinic, after the diagnosis has been established.

3. The person referred back from a specialty clinic for long-term follow-up in a family practice setting.

4. And, in addition, especially at the community center satellite clinic, old persons, frequently seen in a health maintenance program, who are essentially well or coping adequately with controlled chronic illness. They are seen in order to conserve their present good health or to maintain a plateau, with stabilized chronic disease, as long as possible, and perhaps on an organized home care arrangement during the terminal phase of illness.

The family nurse practitioner trainees saw any category of patient, although a real effort was made to keep them away from difficult differential diagnostic problems and close to patients with the major health problems that would be encountered frequently.

Problem-oriented patient records served an essential function in continuity of care, and from the start the Primex students were taught to complete each workup with a problem list and plan, the latter to be suggested by them with collaboration from, and Socratic teaching by, the preceptors. When a flow sheet was indicated, this was the trainee's responsibility—again, the parameters for it were talked over, first, with their preceptors.

Spring, 1972. Much of the psychological approach to the nurse practitioner's content came from my earlier Cornell experience in teaching public health nursing (community health, as it was later termed) to basic undergraduate students who, during one of their senior semesters, combined the theoretical and clinical content of community health and psychiatric nursing.

Life-cycle theory, as projected by Erikson, and psychosocial parameters of stress were introduced as content for Primex. In the latter, major health problems were examined for the impact of life-cycle stages and for the relevance of say, Parad and Caplan's approach to *Crisis in Families* and Suchman's *Stages of Illness.* Suppose the seminar happened to be about tuberculosis in a family. Our conceptual framework would include consideration of needed clinical knowledge, and the behavioral science knowledge required for dealing with dissimilar chronological age and disease stages, situations in which tuberculosis presented itself to more than one family member.

In discussing several hypothetical patients in a seminar, each student would have given thought to one of them in preparation for the session. Each patient (and other family members in the home) would be considered for needed care.

Among the questions to be considered are: What history and clinical findings would one look for? What clues would alert the practitioner to the possibilities? What laboratory studies, and in what order, would be needed? What would the student expect to find? What tuberculin status could be expected in each case? What referrals should be made? What x-ray and culture findings might be observed? What therapy would be indicated and what preventive measures needed for contacts? What measures for monitoring the ongoing progress of the patient and the family contacts? What measures for community control?

These are questions the practitioner was expected to be able both to raise and to answer, focusing on social and economic issues as well as traditional disease control ones.

The students learned from the Parad and Caplan reading, *Crisis in Families,* that the stressful event is, by definition, not solvable in the near future. The problem may overtax the psychological resources of the family. The situation may be a threat to the family's life goals (everything being perceived as "going down the drain"). Tension often rises to a peak and then falls. And the situation often awakens key problems from the near and distant past.

In the Suchman concept, each patient was viewed as moving through certain phases of illness, whether or not these are perceived. Dealing with the person effectively requires awareness of the psychological stage the individual is in.

What is called "the symptom-experiencing stage" tells the patient that "something is wrong."

"The assumption of the sick-role stage" often finds him or her casting about for help. Lay referrals frequently have a high priority. It is in this phase that the patient and/or family recognizes that "I need (or he/she needs) care."

The "care-contact stage" is considered the phase of transition from lay to professional advice, "a search for authoritative sanction to become legitimately ill."

In the "dependent-patient stage," most patients tend to transfer responsibility to the professional and to the significant helping person within the family. This is a period of great receptivity. "Tell me what to do, and I'll do it." But often there is compliance without genuine collaborative participation.

And finally, for those who recover or who reach a rehabilitative plateau, the patient says, through speech or behavior, "I don't need you anymore."

June, 1972. Last weekend, I was at home cleaning my apartment when I heard a horrifying newsflash on the radio: the old Broadway Central Hotel had completely collapsed, disintegrating in a cloud of dust, plaster and marble columns within a few minutes of the initial rumble and the discovery of a cracked wall.

In those few minutes police had successfully evacuated the building. No one was believed to have been inside, although roof, walls and its multiple floors were lying as though an explosion had blown them all into the street. Several hundred welfare residents, most without friends or families, had been left without any possessions except the clothing they had been wearing and they were now standing dazed in the street, waiting for a Red Cross disaster unit which would set up in another welfare hotel to act as a shelter till plans were made for each person for the night. The disaster unit was even now beginning to transport survivors to the other hotel's lobby, where they would be fed while families—if any—were notified.

By coincidence we had just shown a Red Cross training film "The Shelter" to the nurse practitioner students. It had been made to train volunteers for mass disaster rescue work. It made much of the psychological shock and mass apathy likely to affect the victims and the importance of pairing frightened persons, giving each one responsibility for talking to and comforting one another.

I phoned the Red Cross and said that I was a public health nurse who had occasionally worked in that building with students and knew many of the victims. I asked if I could help by joining the disaster unit at the Hotel Bristol as a volunteer.

My respondent doubted that it was necessary, said they already had had a superb response to their emergency calls, but yes, perhaps it might be comforting for frightened people to see a familiar face. I can see the scene clearly now: the hotel lobby with shabby dazed men and women sitting on hastily set-up bridge chairs, Red Cross volunteers passing out sandwiches and coffee, the victims tending to cluster and stare into space. There was an eerie quiet in spite of the traffic outside the door.

Then I saw the Red Cross film come to life and was glad we had used it in class. The victims were being helped to come out of their stupor and to turn to one another and interact. Here we were, a group of volunteer workers, instantly able to provide primary care of a psychological nature on a large scale.

Spring, 1973. Anamarie Shaefer, a graduate of our first Primex program, said of her own application of the role of nurse practitioner to her clientele in the Visiting Nurse Service:

> "The area in which we (the new nurse practitioners) feel we are contributing most to the patient's welfare is in effectually communicating with the doctor—any doctor—in a language that he understands, the condition of the patient. Through taking a very careful health history, doing a systematic examination, recording the data

clearly, and formulating the problems carefully, we provide the basis for more effective communication and
planning. One doctor commented to my colleague (also
a family practitioner), 'I feel that you have been to France
and now we are both speaking French together."'

Spring, 1974. Dr. Barbara Bates' address at the First Primex
graduation was entitled "Twelve Paradoxes." It has become a classic commentary on the risk of trying anything new, however much
it improves upon the old. In the address she warned the nurse
practitioners:

"You will have knowledge and skills not shared by most
nursing faculties or by most nursing supervisors, nor, for that
matter, by medical faculties or physicians with whom you
work (who know little of nursing). In your future work you
may in fact be 'unsupervisable,' (provoking) considerable discomfort in agencies that are accustomed to a supervisory
organization..."

With the graduation of our fourth class it had become clear that
geriatric care was the field most receptive to the nurse practitioner
and the field where unmet patient needs were greatest. Thus, the
next four classes were prepared as geriatric nurse practitioners
instead of family nurse practitioners, while newly instituted programs were preparing other applicants as nurse practitioners for
pediatric and school nurse clientele.

Fall, 1982. A decade later, nurse practitioners are now being
prepared on a master's degree level as nurse clinicians, some of
whom choose primary nursing as their long-term area of care.

I am glad to have been a part of that moment in time when it first became possible to visualize, throughout the nation, the nurse practitioner as the first person from whom patients could seek help (in Suchman's "symptom-experiencing stage") when something goes wrong. It is a wonderfully human kind of nursing practice.

Thinking back on my own role in helping to pioneer this new direction in the field of nursing, I recognize that virtually all my professional life had been a preparation for this assigmnent. The interaction with the medical and related professions in the Comprehensive Care Clinic at Cornell Medical College, the virtually independent role of a public health nurse in Red Hook, the resource-sharing approach to problem solving on the Navajo project, all of these had combined to anticipate some development like the nurse practitioner program. The one missing ingredient for me was formal training in the emerging field of geriatrics. And once again I had been extremely fortunate in getting in on this "ahead of the curve," as politicians would say.

Geriatrics, as a term and as a discipline, came late to medical practice here in the United States. Many European countries participated in the trend before we did. Nowhere had it been more clearly identified and developed as a medical specialty than in the United Kingdom, particularly Scotland.

So I was lucky to have my application for a Fogarty Senior Fellowship approved (the first nurse to be so recognized, I was given to understand) and on the strength of that to be able to spend almost six months during 1976 participating in the field under the tutelage of some of the early pioneers, such as Sir Ferguson Anderson in Glasgow.

When I first returned from Glasgow I had one memorable moment that has to rank with highlights of a 50-year career. One day I chanced to be talking with Dr. Frank Glenn, chief surgeon of New York Hospital and one of the great professors in modern medicine. Dr. Glenn asked me what, if anything, he needed to know that I could tell him about this new field of geriatric medicine.

I said immediately, "Dr. Glenn, we need better thermometers here in the hospital. The ones we have don't measure low enough. And old people, we have learned through observation, have the capacity to stay alive at temperatures lower than any of our thermometers can register." Dr. Glenn saw to it that we got new thermometers for the hospital.

Chapter 9

New Girl at School

I n the summer of 1980, after twenty-nine years on the staff of the Cornell University-New York Hospital School of Nursing as a teacher of Public Health Nursing and later Geriatric Nursing, I retired. For many of these years I had a joint appointment in the Cornell Medical College as a consultant in Public Health Nursing.

I had worked with nearly 2,000 nursing students, a large number of whom went into public health. There was hardly a state I could go to in the country where I couldn't find a public health nursing supervisor or teacher who had been one of my students.

Retirement followed the months of relative inactivity brought on by a stroke. Perhaps inactivity is the wrong term to use; rehabilitation was active indeed, but the effort to regain mobility complicated by loss of peripheral vision was disheartening, as was returning to teaching for a final semester in which I could manage well enough in the classroom, but could not take responsibility for what I loved best, clinical teaching. Clinical teaching in public health settings had always taken the students and me to wherever patients needed care: at the bedside, in the clinic, and especially in the patient's home.

After retiring, still using a walker to get around, I knew I couldn't continue to live in New York City. For one thing, I could not cross a street in the time of one traffic light, and New York is no place to be stuck in the middle of a street when the light changes. I also couldn't carry anything weighing more than several pounds; I wouldn't be able to live as I had, obviously. Going into a nursing home would have been a very poor fit for me. A lifecare community, where I could live in my own apartment, would be ideal. But many such places wouldn't admit me because they didn't think I could manage alone.

I decided to move from New York City to the Life Care Community of Foulkeways at Gwynedd, a Quaker-sponsored development near Philadelphia, where five friends who were former members of the Cornell faculty had preceded me. I had been on the Foulkeways waiting list for a long time prior to the stroke. They took me reluctantly, but it has certainly worked out. I'm better now than when I came.

August 7, 1980. The moving van arrived at nine, and the friends who were driving me from New York City were at the door at ten. My brother, Don, took me from the apartment to the car and said goodbye so fast that the car didn't even need to find a parking space on East 68th Street. It was a hot, sunny day and we had a smooth trip with no traffic holdups, stopping for lunch at the William Penn Inn, across the street from our destination.

The moving van and we entered the gate almost simultaneously. Good friends already in residence here formed an efficient welcoming committee—Ena, Margery, Hendrika, and Mary—all of them pillars at Cornell when I began teaching. They're very protective of me still, "After all, we brought you up from a pup." And in truth, they did. By dinner time the furniture was settled in place and I accompanied Margery to my first dinner in the dining room. Ena elected to help unpack while we were gone, accomplishing the miracle of having some 300 books on bookcase shelves before we returned to a hectic evening of further unpacking and bedmaking.

August 10. The view is lovely. It's like living in a tree house. The studio has a balcony which looks directly into a tall pine tree and through it, at a distance, to the woods. One looks down onto other people's pocket-handkerchief-sized, jewel-like gardens at close range—perhaps a dozen of them are visible between the buildings and the woods.

The apartment entrance, on the side opposite the balcony, is on a sort of aerial walkway much like the deck of an ocean liner, arranged around a grassy quadrangle. The front door, too, if left open with only the screen door closed, looks directly into another treetop. Morning sun enters across the balcony, sunset shows over the aerial walkway. There is a tiny Pullman kitchen, and a large bathroom. Although my apartment—one room—is small, the furniture fits in well and when the pictures and mirrors go up next week, it will be lovely and very homey.

August 12. Seventy-eight acres of thinly-wooded landscape harbors this self-governing hamlet within the larger town of Gwynedd, an old Welsh-Quaker area of families who came over with William Penn. Gwynedd itself has many modern homes today but Foulkeways remains an unspoiled and lovely enclave within it.

A good road surrounds the perimeter of the grounds, with cut-off to small parking lots within reach of each group of houses.

Once you leave the parking lot on foot, the entire community can be travelled without meeting a car. This means that there is a lot of walking done. Everyone who is in individual housing walks. A half-way house and a health center are located where walking is not essential. I have literally walked the rubber tips off my quad cane and had to change them today.

The food is good and attractively served in a large, gracious central dining room, which also takes reservations for guests. Most people take only one meal a day in the dining room, although elderly or fragile residents (or those who simply want to) may take all meals there. The outdoor swimming pool of a nearby Holiday Inn is available to Foulkeways residents for nominal seasonal fee, and the pools of two nearby Y's are used in winter. [In 1988 Foulkeways opened its own excellent indoor pool, which I enjoy immensely.] I've been swimming every day since I arrived, something I thought I'd probably never do again. Many residents have their own cars and are wonderfully hospitable about sharing their extra car space to and from the pool.

August 15. In the dining room and at other public gatherings, at first, people seem quite old and their handicaps show. But as I meet and talk with residents ranging from a low of 65 to age 100, their thinking and range of interests strike me as astonishingly young and flexible; they still look at things with plenty of enthusiasm and wonder.

Of the 350 residents, about two-thirds (individuals or couples) live quite independently in their own well-maintained apartments (studio or one or two bedrooms). Perhaps thirty-two of the remainder have studio apartments in the half-way house, where some assistance is available, if necessary, around the clock. Those who will need skilled nursing care for life, because of degenerative diseases, are in the health care center permanently.

Additional health care beds offer temporary short-term convalescent care to those who are returning from nearby hospitals or who are under observation to see if hospitalization is required. The majority of us will remain in our own apartments for life.

In truth, I'm frightened by the thought that this is forever. That's a wholly new experience, to be in any place that's final, that doesn't have other possibilities coming after it. But perhaps its permanence is like the permanence of my twenty-nine years at Cornell: there's definitely an aspect of continuity to it but there's also the possibility of doing so many kinds of things across the years that richly rewarding variations are present here, too.

August 22. Loving kindness of a sort that I have seen only in exceptional family groups (and perhaps in some communities of nuns) is everywhere: outgoing warmth, personal interest, humor and concern. An enormous amount of voluntary work is done by perhaps one-third of the more vigorous and motivated residents, which is what makes this a community instead of an institution. Serving on some forty resident-organized committees ranging from health center volunteers to hospitality hosts to newspaper reporters and editors, these volunteers have created a village which is a beehive of thoughtful and well-planned action.

Next to the experience of studying and living for a time in Scotland, this appears to be the most democratic land I've found. But it is responsibly democratic, with little rigidity and few rules.

The faces of people, especially some of the oldest Quakers, are remarkable studies of maturity and interest. I knew of, but did not believe that there still were persons alive who routinely used the familiar second person singular personal pronoun without self-consciousness because they have spoken that way all their lives. The telephone rings, "Friend Doris, how does thee do and welcome to Foulkeways. Will thee take dinner with me tomorrow night? I shall ask two others to meet thee."

Not more than one in eight or nine residents is a member of the religious Society of Friends, but board members are Quakers and Foulkeways was originally created by the Gwynedd Monthly Meeting of Friends. Their philosophy permeates the life style of this community, which is without a particular religious persuasion.

Minority groups of all kinds seem underrepresented but they are certainly here among us. I am conspicuously young—the new girl at school. Everyone has been both welcoming and protective during this orientation period. My calendar is full of dinner dates for the next two weeks.

Each day is very full for everyone, but it is up to the individual resident to decide how involved he or she wants to be. There are only two unforgivable sins: to appear at anyone's doorway without first phoning or having an invitation, and phoning a neighbor during "privacy hours," before nine a.m. or from one to three in the afternoon. I don't mean that no one is about at those times; the scene is fairly active, but it is up to the individual to decide whether to be out or to withdraw.

September 20. Two interesting brief job opportunities have suddenly appeared: reviewing the gerontological and geriatric texts and references published in 1980 (and judging the "Books of the Year Awards in Geriatric Nursing") for the *American Journal of Nursing* and an invitation to give the keynote address at the White House Miniconference on Aging in San Diego.

I hope that out of this miniconference will come recommendations reaching out to the delegates to next year's White House Conference on Aging, which will pave the way for using more of the knowledge we already have by getting it out of the literature and into practice. [Unfortunately, this did not happen.]

The thrust has to be toward educating our citizenry about the normal developmental process of becoming older, to enable people to anticipate normal changes of aging and to differentiate between being old and having pathology—illness—superimposed on aging.

Two crisis states of older persons that receive far too little attention, it seems to me, are failure of confidence (often following a relatively minor incident) and reactive depression (following multiple losses so closely spaced that the old person has had little or no time to work them through by proper grieving before another loss occurs). We also need increased comprehension of Alzheimer's disease, and multi-infarct dementia. One of the most important pieces of knowledge to be accepted by the laity—as well as by professionals—is that these diseases are not simply consequences of growing older.

Professionals must also focus on the reversible forms of brain failure, those rapid-onset conditions which, left undiagnosed and untreated, or wrongly treated, bring unnecessary despair and disruption of life to the victim and family members.

We already know more about the strategies for coping with chronic brain failure—simple environmental management strategies —than we are using with most patients today. A nurse named Irene Burnside and a good many other nurses and social workers have produced a continuous flow of practical information about the effective daily management of confused and brain-failed persons, individually and in groups, in various settings.

But diagnostic techniques for chronic brain failure are still surprisingly primitive. Why? And treatment is only palliative. From

Great Britain and from some experiments here, for example, at the Burke Rehabilitation Center in Westchester County, New York, we are seeing that day care programs can contribute a good deal to the lives of chronically brain-failed persons and their families.

April 30, 1981. The time of Christmas until Easter was a period of reaching out, taking on new types of volunteer work, finishing some writing, having several pieces of work in print (among them an article in *Yankee* Magazine and an editorial in a recent issue of *The American Nurse*. Each of these produced a small snowstorm of mail: the first from ex-patients and colleagues of World War II Army Nurse Corps days, the latter from students and colleagues at Cornell.

A few Foulkeways residents have part-time jobs away from here and many more are busy with volunteer work, some as far away as Philadelphia or in their former home communities. But the largest number are volunteers in community activities here at Foulkeways. I have begun to work with seventy-five other volunteers in the health center, doing things with those of our neighbors who are no longer able to be independent.

We do small things. I do reading once a month for people who can't read and I write oral histories for people who, because of blindness, deafness or something else, are out of communication-with their families. For instance, a woman who can't hear or talk with her relatives on the phone can write a story about her life that will be passed on to them. Mary is her name and as she dictated to me, in fragments, her childhood memories, this summary of herself came out whole and clear. Another deeply confused lady, often no longer able to think rationally, still makes perceptive comments at times. One example: "She was a newspaper woman. Her writing was objective. She always checked her facts."

March 11, 1982. The cover of my new co-authored textbook arrived from England, where it is being published. Written with Sir Ferguson Anderson, Francis Caird and Robin Kennedy, with whom I had spent my 1976 sabbatical working in Glasgow, it is titled *Gerontology and Geriatric Nursing*. It will be published in October.

A concatenation of happy circumstances has resulted in my part-time appointment to the Geriatric Nursing faculty at the University of Pennsylvania, an experience which I am enjoying very much. Other brief, part-time work opportunities have occurred with the Commonwealth Fund and the Robert Wood Johnson Foundation.

In a project called the Living-at-Home Program, the Commonwealth Fund and associated foundations are giving ten or twelve localities with high proportions of low-income elderly the money to coordinate service organizations into a single case-management process. Many of the fragile elderly and disabled who wish to do so will be able to remain in their own homes instead of going into nursing homes.

Also, this is about a report which I did before I retired, which was supposed to be published and wasn't. Seems the National League for Nursing published it but never told me, I suppose figuring that anyone who'd had a stroke and was living in a lifecare community wouldn't know. One of my University of Pennsylvania students met me in a hall at school and told me what an interesting project it must have been "when you visited those seventeen universities and did that follow-up study on faculty research."

"How did you hear about that?" I asked her, thinking she was some kind of clairvoyant. And she told me it had been published and that she had read it in the library.

Presently, I feel that I've moved from being fully retired to being not quite retired—a very nice feeling indeed!

October 20, 1985. A pleasant custom at the University of Pennsylvania Nursing School is the "brown bag lunch." This is an informal lunch time seminar, requested and arranged by students. Last Thursday I was asked to do one on the use of restraints.

I sat at the head of the table and began to talk. There were about sixteen people listening to me. Then a student and a teacher came in, carrying a restraint. The student held the restraint while the teacher sat down next to me and said very seriously, yet loud enough for the whole class to hear:

"Doris, the facility is very concerned about you. You've been very confused for the last three weeks. Your thinking isn't clear and we've had complaints from the Police Department that you've been wandering back and forth in an erratic way between 30th Street Station and the school."

She said it gently, very caringly. The expression on those sixteen faces changed. After all, that particular teacher is not a person who jokes.

She said, "We do want you to finish this class you've started. But we think that you ought to have a safe jacket on so that you don't fall out of your chair. Your balance is very, very poor. You would be safer with the jacket on."

We'd planned all of this, of course, and I had carefully memorized all the protests that I could find in the literature about restrained patients.

So I protested as hard as I could protest. (We had agreed beforehand that I would not struggle physically against the restraint but would make it as difficult verbally as I could.) I made quite a racket.

At some point the students gradually realized that this was a role play. But under restraints I continued to teach a suddenly serious class. It was the same content I would have given if I were lecturing unimpeded. I recognized that all through the class the students were very uncomfortable.

I don't believe I taught that class any differently because I was being restrained. But at the end of it, the student responses were wonderful. They had recognized, for the first time in their lives (these were all experienced nurses), that when someone is being restrained the nurses don't want to look at the victim.

One said, "I was distancing myself as hard as I could from you. I couldn't bear the sight of you in that restraint."

Well, if she felt that troubled, it must have been a great class. Another student said, "All the things that you cried out in protest had a thread of continuity through them."

And it was true. They were very different kinds of comments: "Bring me a hammer! Bring me scissors!" I even tried to bribe them. I said, "I'll give you five dollars if you take this jacket off me!"

But the student said that every one of the things I had yelled out had a connection; all of them simply were saying, "Please don't treat me this way."

January 1986. I have learned much from fellow residents at Foulkeways about what the chronically-ill elderly want and can use in their later years. One of them told me:

"We want to continue as we always were. Some of us want to live in groups, some of us wish to live alone. Some in cities, some in the country. Some of us extend ourselves easily, some of us are loners and in the late seventies, eighties and nineties we're not going to change the habits of a lifetime. Some of us prefer the cultural groups we're used to, some find it adventurous to mix with different cultures and make new friends, to have friendships that start when we're really old. Some of us like books and theatre and some like the handwork sort of hobbies. Some of us like to swim or fish or garden. Some like to be with children. Let us just follow our own interests without being typed as old. Let us keep on being ourselves! Don't you do our deciding for us."

Many Foulkeways residents contributed to the comments which follow. In particular I am indebted to Ena Fisher for the concern and sensitivity which she brought to these discussions out of her experience as a nurse before her retirement as well as from her activity here as a Foulkeways resident.

Some of the voices which were raised said the following:

"There are many ways you who are younger can help. You can help enact laws providing care in long-term illness, provide settings that relieve us of unnecessary worry, that give us reasonable freedom from fear of financial crises, with assurance of care when in need. And good human relationships throughout that care. Some of us do better when we know there's help around the clock, if we need it; some of us do best in our own homes and we'd rather take care of ourselves as long as we can. If we're alone and sick at home, we need to know that help is there if we have to get it."

"Don't desert us. We're prepared to contribute our own finances as long as we have an income. But whether we worked and saved, inherited, or are entirely supported by Social Security, we need to know that in sickness the same standards of care are going to be there: no greater privilege, and no less. We want and need independence from our families but we want them to remain interested and to care. In the absence of any family members we want someone nearby to care about, even more than we want someone to care about us. That's part of the meaning of living, isn't it? We still want to be in touch with children and young people. We want them to understand that being old is not being different, that everybody who lives long enough, even a new baby, is going to be old one day."

"We're pretty realistic. We know that no organized human help is going to reverse what we've lost. It's not going to bring back our spouses, our friends, our physical strength or our youth."

"What can we give? Probably not as much, each one of us, as we ever did, in service and in socialization, although with more spare time and good community organization, some of us still will give a lot."

"Have you who are planning for our care, the care of the entire aged population, ever been in the skilled-nursing homes and halfway houses of the best of our life-care communities? Have you seen the practice of loving and respect there? The gracious living? Their ways of keeping us comfortable in long-term illness? And keeping us peaceful, as we die? You would see people who are irreversibly ill but attractively dressed, hair neatly coiffed, comfortably seated in a chair if we cannot walk, perhaps not able to get up to greet you with a handshake and words, but often with a smile on our lips or in our eyes. We, the old long-term patients, know that you care, offering us your presence. Perhaps our neighbors and friends do not stay for long visits—it may hurt them too much. But they come, as family substitutes, showing their concern, showing that we matter, watering our plants, reading to those of us who can't see, bringing our mail, taking us out on the terrace on a warm, sunny day."

These are small, simple things not exclusive to a skilled nursing facility or a good half-way house. Any caring group that organizes itself could do these simple things for its home-bound or institutionalized elderly. But the network, the mesh into which both the needs and the helping services are woven, has to be as organized and as continuously available through a telephone and a human help-line as it is in our Foulkeways community, with a melding of well-directed professional, administrative and volunteer staff. It cannot be fragmented and still work and it cannot be rigid.

I and my fellow residents, most of us living actively and independently, and some of us needing moderate to total care, have the assurance that we will get the help we need from both the administration and from our fellow residents. Not just help for our physical needs, but with our mental health as well. We are privileged and we know it. We are trying to plough back into the community the compassionate philosophy of caring that we see around us.

One comment from an old and frail but very active resident is typical of the thinking that is reflected here daily:

"You hear many old people say that the world only values material things today. I don't think that is true. Both people and things are important if you're going to grow old well. When you care about things and you use people, old age is going to be heavy, overwhelming. But if you care about people and you use things, you can take a lot of the losses of chronic illness and still stay strong. You can reach out and be reached."

No one kind of program, day care, nursing home, home care, is going to be the right answer for everyone. The chronically-ill elderly need options, all of them imaginative, all of them well-run.

I had the chance to say something like the above when I was invited to testify before the United States Senate's Committee on Aging, chaired by Senator John Heinz, in May of 1983. Unfortunately, I was limited to five minutes and asked to speak only about legislation that might offer protection against financial abuse of the elderly. Had I been given more time, I like to think I would have made a plea against the emotional neglect of the elderly as well. I like to think that the senators present that day really would have listened and that by 1990 there truly would be a nation-wide commitment to the kind of treatment that all people deserve in declining age.

Well, it has not happened in 1990. But some day, please God, let it be so.

Chapter 10

To the Great Wall of China

It was an adventure of a lifetime in 1986—participation in a People-to-People Foundation delegation to China as part of a group of American nurses who were guests of the China Medical Association and the China Nurses Association. We brought a traveling workshop to, and learned from, Chinese nurses in Beijing, Nanjing and Hangchou.

It seems clear that by whatever means my name got included on the invitational list, the fact that I had both visual and ambulatory problems was unknown to the Foundation. When I replied to the invitation saying that such a trip was out of the question for me, they indicated astonishment at their own lack of awareness. By that time I had become excited at the very thought of going along. Encouraged by fellow residents and Foulkeways' own nurse practitioners, I agreed that if the delegation were willing to take the risk of having me, I was willing to be their fifteenth delegate. So I represented the field of geriatric nursing and offered a living example of geriatric care.

On that basis (with the help of younger colleagues, whose eyes and arms I often needed) I traveled to China, enjoying it immensely. I promptly fell in love with the Chinese people, visited hospitals devoted both to Western type and to traditional medical care, went to the Great Wall (which I was unable to climb), the Ming tombs, the Forbidden City, and I journeyed all day by train through farm country and admired China's beautiful babies. (A friend once commented, "Oriental babies look so *finished*." Indeed they do.)

I will always be glad that I saw China during this mid-1980s political thaw in relations between our two countries. Although on the trip I sometimes found my mind making promises that my body couldn't keep, both my colleagues and I agreed that I had managed pretty well.

Our interaction with Chinese nurse colleagues went far beyond my expectations. It was immensely satisfying on both sides. Once in a park in Hangchou I rested under a tree, being unable to keep up with the others on one of China's endless walks. I spent the time talking with our interpreter, a young Chinise nurse who had had a year's training as a medical translator in the United States.

This helped her translate for American consultants in medicine and in nursing when they visited China on official business. I casually mentioned something about a Navajo Indian patient I once had. She replied enthusiastically, "Oh, I know about the Navajo. My American mentor used to work with them."

There are more than one billion Chinese people and I had landed under a tree in a Chinese park with the one Chinese student who, like myself, had had Dr. Kurt Duschle for a mentor. How is that for a coincidence? Despite the wide differences in our age, culture, and experience, we both admired the same things about Kurt as a teacher and a friend.

All China seems to be on the move, with rebuilding going on everywhere. Everyone works very hard, with immense vitality. Millions of bicycles were in motion, cycling with orderliness and dignity, spaced so carefully that each one appears to be buffered from the others.

In cities that are incredibly crowded at home, at work, and on the street, this spacing of bicycles is very arresting. When I mention it to nurses and doctors, their explanation is, "A bicycle is the only place one can ever be alone. I love to ride to work and home again." Nowhere else before had the notion of solitude on a bicycle been pointed out to me, although I instantly recognized it as true.

"Check with my supervisor" seems to be a key phrase in the vocabulary of the Chinese people at the time of our visit. In spite of the individual friendliness of the people, they seem to have little sense of independence. Even the smallest request, if it deviates from routine, is answered, "I will have to check with my supervisor first."

This is still an autocratic, if newly benign, government. It is one in which persons who apparently have considerable low-level responsibility cannot make any independent decisions. The words "relationship" and "contact"—which everyone seemed eager to engage in—seemed to me to be used interchangeably.

Later I came to realize that "contact" was only used to describe an interaction with a person who might help the speaker with some personal gain (whether it be job, housing, assignment within a place of employment, hours of work, or some other advantage), while "relationship" denoted friendliness and enjoyment in what was frequently only a single interaction with someone who might never again be encountered. When "relationship" was used to describe our meetings with Chinese professionals, it implied something more like pleasure than practicality, even if it did add to their knowledge while giving them a chance to practice their English.

It was a great joy to visit the famous Peking Union Medical College Hospital and School of Nursing, where so many of my own American teachers had once taught. It is still a superior institution. I met an elderly nurse, Mme. Yun-Zhu She, whom I had heard about for more than forty years. She had been at New York Hospital in 1934 as a Rockefeller Foundation fellow in nursing. Only two years ago I learned from a visiting Chinese scholar at the University of Pennsylvania that she was alive and lived in Tianjin.

We began to correspond. Although she is now retired and living in a city which our delegation did not visit, she traveled all the way to Beijing with the vice-president of her hospital to spend one evening with me. It was a wonderful evening, in which I learned more about Chinese nursing under the present regime than I did from all the other nurses with whom I spoke. We will continue to correspond.

When the 15 members of our delegation first were accepted, each of us was asked to prepare abstracts of class content which we might teach Chinese nurses, if requested. These were winnowed down to about 45 topics. We were then asked to send written notes for three class sessions each, so that our interpreters in China could familiarize themselves with the translations they would be called upon to perform. Nurses in each city we visited had the chance to select which topics they especially wanted to hear from the 45-course menu. For my own talks I tried to keep to very basic issues of geriatric nursing care—ideas on health maintenance while growing older and on treatment when illness was superimposed on normal aging.

On arrival in each city, we were met at the airport or train station by medical and nursing officials and it was then we first learned what our schedule would be and what topics were desired. Each city provided its own bus and driver, guides and interpreters. The latter were either students or young graduate nurses, whose English varied widely. One young nurse, employed as a translator by the China Medical Association, accompanied us all the time we were in China. She was really a fluent translator.

Most days began with 7 o'clock breakfast. By 7:45 our bus left for a sightseeing trip, often poetically titled. Example:"Viewing goldfish on West Lake at Three Pools Reflecting the Moon and Stars." This involved a ride through the city while thousands of citizens were cycling to work, a short ferry ride across West Lake to a beautiful park, then a 15-minute walk over a scenic trail to "Three Pools Reflecting the Moon and Stars."

Hundreds of tourists from many lands (the largest number from Japan) were moving along the trail or could be seen on boats. Even larger numbers of Chinese were in the park: schoolchildren there for an outing, families on their one-day-a-week holiday, bus loads of farmers and workers from all over China who had been given a reward for exceeding production quotas.

By 10 a.m. we usually were at a hospital where a gracious welcome was given by top staff officials. Then with several medical students or student nurses accompanying us, each of us visited different hospital wards and treatment rooms. We were permitted to see patient records and have the parts we were especially interested in translated for us. Most of the patients were on long, open wards—as had been true in many American hospitals when I was a student nurse.

Chinese doctors and nurses were not without understanding of modern techniques, yet a large hospital might have only one four-bed intensive-care unit for all its surgical patients, and another three or four beds in the medical wards equipped for cardiac monitoring. An enormous increase in hospitals, professional staff training and technology will be needed if one billion people are to profit from today's potential for health care.

Considering the poverty and constraints from the cultural revolution, China used what small budget it had for health care to improve the nutrition of an entire population, to immunize against major communicable threats, and to set its health priorities in ways that most public health personnel would approve. Its plans for the next two decades sound encouraging. It was sad to learn that the United States was withdrawing its World Health Organization (W.H.O.) payments because China has been using a considerable part of its W.H.O. benefits for population control. The U.S.A. still will not pemit its money to be used for such a purpose.

Health training during the cultural revolution was almost nil. Most doctors in traditional hospitals of Oriental medicine now have some knowledge of Western medicine as well. Today's graduates of the traditional medical schools are taking parts of their internships in Western-type hospitals. Yet adequate care of one billion people, given present restraints and lack of hard currency to purchase technological equipment, truly is restricted.

The nurses I observed and talked with are fine, decent people, struggling to hold on to ideals of good patient care. Yet nursing is at the bottom of the ladder of power, influence, status, and money in health care—as it was for so long in America. Both nurses and doctors, as well as the non-professional staff, are assigned to hospitals by government bureaus which appeared to us to lack sensitivity for matching staff to patient needs in a particular setting.

Hospital workers today (perhaps Chinese workers of every type) have great patience and the hope of a life better than anything they have previously known. The cultural revolution, however, destroyed much that was good in hospitals by its closing of the best medical and nursing schools for a period of ten years and by its banishment of their intellectual leaders to menial jobs. Even today, however, to get any standard procedure changed the worker (including a supervisor) must appeal to the unit which is the individual's source of authority. Such appeals are necessary to approve a job change, to enroll in further education, to obtain new equipment, or to improve staffing patterns. Hospital directors, directors of nursing and head nurses were all quite frank in discussing the limitations this process imposed upon them.

It is difficult to express the ambivalence with which our delegation and I personally reacted during almost every hour of our multiple hospital visitations. On one hand, there were the hopeful signs of the recent open-door policy and the fact that Western professional groups like ours were indeed being welcomed. There were the continuous announcements from party leaders that rigid Marxist doctrines were being re-examined.

There seems to be work for everyone with health care preparation. Everyone looked clean, well fed, healthy and comfortably dressed. Everyone seemed cheerful, especially with their peers and with children. Doctors and nurses met were intellectually curious and deeply concerned with patient care.

We did not detect discontent, even though we looked for it in talking with patients and their families. Admittedly, we saw only the wards that our hosts wanted to show us, but once on a ward we were free to talk, via a translator, with any patient or staff member. No Chinese wanted to talk about the cultural revolution; questions are always answered with standard criticism of the "Gang of Four."

Yet obviously that movement, which was so damaging to people, places, and values, was broader and deeper than any "Gang of

Four." It cannot easily be removed as an influence. One has to wonder, looking at the great group of workers now in their twenties, who among them had been those teenage Red Guards and now are parents of China's one-child families? What values are they really passing along to their own children?

The cultural revolution seems to be entirely over. Musicians, artists, craftsmen, and scholars are again recognized as people and are working hard to forge a new and freer China. But the forces that created both the strengths and problems of China are all here among these billion citizens.

Like the nurses whom we observed and to whom we taught classes each afternoon, I can hope. To make a slight inroad on their paucity of information about our modern work in geriatric nursing, I have pledged myself for the next academic year to spend one day each month scanning the new geriatric literature and duplicating material which nurses at Peking Union Medical College and at Tanjin's First Central Hospital may find useful to translate and make available.

Nine days a year to help build a geriatric nursing library from scratch seems a puny handful of building blocks. But our Chinese friends seemed to find it meaningful, whether practically or psychologically I honestly don't know. (Their letters acknowledging receipt of material have been warm and grateful. One of them wrote me a fascinating comment. She said, "A good example is a silent order.")

In the evenings after work we attended theater, gymnastic exhibitions, walked in the crowded streets. In each city we were given a banquet by our Chinese counterparts. There were endless toasts of good wishes: to our countries and their people, to better care for patients, to world peace, to better doctor-nurse relationships, to friendship. The younger nurses usually put on a skit of hospital life; no fluency of language was needed to appreciate the pantomime. Then one of the Chinese would approach an American with a microphone. "Sing song for China, please."

I said that I could not sing—and believe me, that's the truth. I said I did not know any songs.

"Oh, yes, you know song. Sing about American lady wears fish box on feet."

"American lady wears fish box? I never heard of such a song."

"Oh, Doris, You know song. Everybody knows. American lady with feet size nine wears herring boxes without topsis instead of sandals."

"Oh, you mean 'Clementine.'"

"Sing 'Clementine' for China, please."

I think that was my unforgettable moment of truth. Whatever am I doing here? This naive, altruistic American nurse who traveled half-way around the world to introduce sophisticated gerontology and geriatric nursing to China, and what do they really want from me? To hear me belt out "Clementine" in a Chinese restaurant!

There were other non-professional moments that were more serious and also more memorable. I was in China on three Sundays, during two of which we were in transit from one city to another. On the middle Sunday, in Nanjing, a sightseeing trip was planned.

I wanted to get a relationship with Chinese Christians to find out how they were surviving. Churches had been reopened in 1980 after more than thirty years of enforced closure. I knew that an enormous amount of liberal arts and science education, along with Western medical care, had entered China prior to the 1940s by way of Christian missionaries' schools. I wondered if there was any evidence of this remaining in 1986.

I went to the desk of the hotel at which we were staying and spoke to the assistant manager. "Is there a Christian church open now in Nanjing?"

"Yes, madam, it reopened in 1980."

"I would like to go to the service there today. Is it in this part of the city?"

"Yes, madam, it is not far from this hotel. But you would not wish to attend service there. You would see no Chinese, only visitors from other countries. We have a very fine trip for your delegation today. The bus will go at half past eight."

"I know there is a trip," I said. "My colleagues will all go on it. But I wish to attend the Christian church. Could I get a taxi?"

"We will take your delegation to Sun Yat Sen's tomb this morning. You will not want to miss that."

"Thank you. I know today's trip will be very interesting. But I would like to go to the Christian church."

"Please come back in 15 minutes. I will have to check with my supervisor."

When I returned I was told, "Madam, we have arranged everything you wish for you. The bus will stop at the Christian church for 10 minutes so that all of you can take pictures there."

"Thank you. But I think I did not make myself clear. I wish to go to the service of the Christian church while my colleagues take this morning's sightseeing trip. Can you send a taxi to pick me up after church to return me here for lunch with the group?"

"The bus will stop at the Christian church."

Indeed the church was close to the hotel. The bus stopped. We all got out, walked down an alley and entered a large traditional

Protestant church whose interior was neatly painted. Nicely-bound new red hymn books were in the pews—printed in Chinese, of course. There were new attractive ceiling lights. And there were two pulpits, one occupied by a male preacher, the other by a woman.

The congregation—perhaps fifty or sixty people in the front pews—was singing a familiar hymn, "Morning Has Broken," in Chinese. This was followed by several other traditional hymns, or at least hymns with traditional tunes. Scattered through the church were perhaps another hundred people of all ages, some of whom were adolescents, both girls and boys. We sat for a few moments. Our guide appeared at the end of the pew. "Come, we go now." My fellow nurses, who knew that I intended to stay, filed out.

The guide and bus driver returned. "Please, you must go. The bus has to leave soon."

"No. I am not going with you. The hotel manager knows that. If you can stop on your way back to pick me up, it would be nice. Otherwise the hotel manager will send a taxi for me."

The driver and guide, looking troubled, sat down on either side of me. "We cannot leave you."

I said again that the hotel manager understood. Finally they went out politely, but I know they thought poorly of this crazy, stubborn American woman.

A few minutes later I learned that what I had thought was the regular church service turned out to have been a choir rehearsal. Then hundreds of Chinese people poured into the church until every seat was filled and small camp chairs had to be set up in the aisles. The service seemed to be a traditional Protestant one. The hymn tunes were those usually found in a Methodist or Presbyterian hymnal. The woman preacher delivered a fiery sermon in a strong voice. No offering was collected. At the close of the service the hundreds of persons simply vanished.

Just after the driver and guide had left, a young man who evidently had heard our interchange moved to sit near me. "I recognize you," he whispered in English. "I work at your hotel. If you wish, I will walk back with you when church is over." He remained in the rapidly filling pew. I thanked him. A few minutes later an elderly man with a sad lined face approached the pew. The young man looked at him respectfully, seemed to understand the other man's unspoken wishes, gave him his seat and disappeared. The old man sat beside me.

When the service was about to start he turned to me and spoke in a sad, quiet voice. "Before the liberation I was the pastor of this church. I welcome you and thank you for coming this morning." He said no more but participated in the readings and the singing, and listened attentively to the sermon. At the close of the service he said, "Stay here. I will call a taxi and come back." He returned shortly to the now almost empty church. "Come, we will sit near the door and watch for your taxi. I will stay with you until it comes."

We sat and he told me, very carefully, a little about the church, about himself. "I am an ordained Presbyterian minister of missionary training. But I am no longer permitted to preach, only to be an attender of the church. There are several thousand members; about one-fourth come to the service each Sunday. I attend regularly since it was reopened in 1980." He wrote his name for me in Chinese and in English. He spoke of the great variety of activities the church had had prior to its closing. "Now it is only unlocked for two hours each week for choir rehearsal and service."

Young people as they left spoke to him respectfully. He seemed like a defeated old man, yet as I looked I realized that perhaps he was not any older than I. He said, almost imploringly, "Do you believe in God?" And in that moment I thought, "This is not a pastor asking a routine question of a parishioner, nor a missionary seeking a potential convert. This is a man asking for assurance." I felt it strongly.

I replied, "I want to answer your question with a beautiful quotation that was found scratched on a wall in a cellar in Germany where Jews had been hidden from the Nazis. It is what I too believe. 'I believe in the sun, even when it is not shining. I believe in love, even when not feeling it. I believe in God, even when he is silent.'"

The pastor of long ago reached out and took both my hands and we sat like that for a couple of minutes without speaking. When I looked up, tears were running down his cheeks. He made no attempt to wipe them away. He still had tears when the taxi came. He blessed me and I went away, almost surely never to see each other again. He has my card. I have his name and address,and I will write him. I think these few minutes will stay with each of us forever.

Our days in Nanjing have been much more genuinely spontaneous than the time in Beijing—less carefully structured and wonderfully open during the hospital visits. Using student doctors and nurses as interpreters, we have been encouraged to visit wards randomly, to talk with patients and patients' families, to pick up patients' charts for translation.

The staff takes great pride in their work, records are well kept, and there are good nursing-care plans on some if not all records. Acupuncture (done by nurses) is used extensively when prescribed, and finger pressure at acupuncture points is taught to patients for self-care or taught to family members who will become caregivers. I have seen this used for the relief of pain, for neurological pathology (Parkinson's disease, for example), for sleeplessness and headache—the points and timing varying with the medical problem.

All the hospitals which we saw, whether Western-type medicine or traditional Chinese, had enormous outpatient facilities. Home care programs are limited to small numbers of far-advanced chronically-ill patients who have been discharged from hospitals. There are no community health nursing services such as our Visiting Nurse organizations, although hospital nurses do make some home visits. All hospitals are understaffed; in medical wards patients help patients as in our old Blockley and Bellevue Hospital wards.

Easy rapport exists between doctors and nurses; head nurses have the authority of British head nurses in the pre-World War II era. Salaries are low but head nurses receive an amount equal to some staff physicians. The director of nursing, with rank and pay equal to that of the assistant director of the hospital, has real internal decision-making capability but no external influence. Nursing school faculty members divide responsibilities between teaching and nursing service. However, student nurses are becoming increasingly difficult to recruit. Young graduates of senior high schools want computer or other office work. Those completing lower high school (equivalent to a 10th grade level) find that their education now can lead to a nursing career.

In the hospitals we visited, I.V. and transfusions were frequently seen but no kidney dialysis units were observed. Chinese-made pacemakers are in use. Antibiotics were available. Drug names, when translated, were mostly unfamiliar to the American nurses. Patients appeared to be quite proud of the care they were receiving. Nurses checking respiration stand at the foot of a bed and mimic the patient's breathing "to recognize when the patient is having difficulty breathing," we were told. The technique of inching a stethoscope across a patient's chest (which I had thought was strictly an American procedure) was used frequently by Chinese doctors.

Some hospitals use both Oriental medicine and Western-type treatment, though usually performed by different doctors. While there are said to be only thirty-eight traditional medical and nursing schools in all of China, many graduates of Western nursing schools work in hospitals that practice traditional Oriental medicine, perhaps because the government is responsible for staffing all hospitals.

Summing up our final workshop, each city successively has seemed less crowded, more beautiful, and conducive to easier relationships with our counterparts. Why we found Hangchou producing more conversational intimacy and intellectual curiosity among both doctors and nurses is hard to explain. We are giving the same papers, the same classes, yet the response is far more exciting.

Perhaps our delegation's reputation for being comfortable to have around is traveling ahead of us. Both we and our hosts seemed less at ease in Beijing when we first reached China. Possibly now both of us know what to expect and therefore are more relaxed. It seems every free moment in the hospitals and classrooms now is filled with the buzz of animated talk—in spite of language difficulties. The exact same classes are more enthusiastically received and discussed. Nurses from both cultures have become like old friends. The atmosphere of adventure and expectation in our relationships is at a peak here in Hangchou and all of us are experiencing more laughter and lightness of heart. It is a good way to end our trip.

Whatever the reasons for the gradual strengthening of relationships between our American delegation and our Chinese hosts, it interests me to see a parallel with my previous professional experiences, both at home and in other countries. Wherever I have worked, the more I get to know the people around me (nurses, doctors, social workers, hospital and health agency administrators, and, of course, patients and their families), the more the artificial barriers that divide and separate seem to be lowered.

When I returned to the United States in September of 1986, it was my hope that the people of these two great nations—China and America—would continue to collaborate, along with their governments, on such issues as the people's health. It seemed reasonable to believe that other mutual concerns would follow: the affirmation of fundamental human rights, the promotion of social progress, the practice of toleration of differences, the goal of abolition of war as a means of settling disputes. I had seen at first-hand how American and Chinese nurses could work together toward not only mutual learning but mutual affection.

Nursing's own international professional organization, the International Council of Nurses, began in the last years of the 19th Century. As such, it was the oldest international professional organization, preceding similar groups representing the fields of medicine, law, and engineering. I deeply desired to see China's nurses return to full membership in the I.C.N., bringing my colleagues from the People's Republic of China back to an organization in which they too were once proud members—to an organization whose members were equally proud of them.

Despite the horrors of Tienanmen Square, I still have faith in the goals I held back in 1986. I have stayed in touch with my Chinese colleagues by letter and by an exchange of teaching materials. It was in reply to my sending a copy of a gerontological nursing textbook that I received a letter in the spring of 1990, beautifully printed in careful English that began, "Dear Teacher." I am touched by the thought that one brief encounter four years ago in a foreign land still evokes such an honorable salutation.

Afterword

nother whole volume could easily have been filled with stories of people and places I wish could have been included, particularly, the exceptional nursing opportunities during the Cornell years. In particular, I would like to mention two non-nursing colleagues there. Alice Ullman (a social worker) and Dr. Mary Goss (a sociologist). I worked with both of them on almost a daily basis through most of those twenty-nine years. They expanded my knowledge of their disciplines and helped me to improve the practice of my own.

A few other events not described in the book include the following: Back in the 1960s I spent one summer at the then U.S. Public Health Service's Communicable Disease Center in Atlanta taking a fine course in Epidemiology, which subject I would later teach. For one entire scholastic year I was "loaned" to the State of Ohio's Health Department in order to gain experience which our nursing school needed, while helping the Ohio Health Department plan expanded rural public health nursing services when the Medicare program began. In the 1970s, on sabbatical leave at the end of twenty-five years at Cornell, I spent time in Scotland studying with Sir Ferguson Anderson, the world's first professor of geriatric medicine.

After retiring from Cornell and moving to Foulkeways in 1980, I spent nine unforgettable years of part-time association with the

School of Nursing a the University of Pennsylvania as a Senior Fellow. In this setting, my own rehabilitation from a stroke was actively promoted by the faculty of Geriatric Nursing (particularly Mathy Mezey and Neville Strumpf) and by the School of Nursing's Dean Claire Fagin.

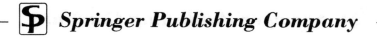
Springer Publishing Company

EXPERTISE IN NURSING PRACTICE
Caring, Clinical Judgement, and Ethics

Patricia Benner, RN, PhD, FAAN, **Christine A. Tanner,** RN, PhD, FAAN, **Catherine A. Chesla,** RN, DNSc; contributions by **Hubert L. Dreyfus,** PhD, **Stuart E. Dreyfus,** PhD and **Jane Rubin,** PhD

The long-awaited sequel to Benner's earlier book, *From Novice to Expert,* this book further analyzes and examines the nature of clinical knowledge and judgement, using the authors' major new research study as its base. The authors interviewed and observed the practice of 130 hospital nurses, mainly in critical care, over a six year period, collecting hundreds of clinical narratives from which they have refined and deepened their explanation of the stages of clinical skill acquisition and the components of expert practice.

Contents:

1995   416pp   0-8261-8700-5   hardcover

536 Broadway, New York, NY 10012-3955 • (212) 431-4370 • Fax (212) 941-7842

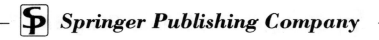
Springer Publishing Company

WHAT EVERY HOME HEALTH NURSE NEEDS TO KNOW
A Book of Readings

Marjorie McHann, RN, Editor

An anthology of practical, up-to-date readings on home care nursing from leading journals, books, and other sources. Readings were selected for their immediate usefulness to clinicians on topics such as medicare coverage, skilled documentation, clinical management, patient education, quality assurance, and legal issues. A valuable resource for students, practicing nurses, and home care administrators.

> **What Every
> Home Health Nurse
> Needs to Know**
> *A Book of Readings*
>
> Marjorie McHann

Partial Contents:

Medicare Coverage Issues • Management and Evaluation • The Denial Dilemma • **Skilled Documentation** • Charting that Makes it through the Medicare Maze • Visit Notes • **Clinical Management** • Productivity • Discharge Planning
Patient Education • Successful Client Teaching — What Makes the Difference? • Helping Older Learners Learn • **Quality Assurance Issues** • Patient Complaints • How to Promote Patient Satisfaction • **Legal Issues** • Legal Implications of Home Health Care • Avoiding Professional Negligence: A Review

1995   210pp   0-8261-9130-4   hardcover

536 Broadway, New York, NY 10012-3955 • (212) 431-4370 • Fax (212) 941-7842

Springer Publishing Company

ADVANCING NURSING EDUCATION WORLDWIDE

Doris Modly, RN, PhD,
Renzo Zanotti, IP, AFD, PhD (C),
Dott. **Piera Poletti, & Joyce J. Fitzpatrick,** RN,
PhD, FAAN, Editors

The purpose of the book is to describe global trends in nursing education, share innovative approaches to it, report and develop cross-cultural and collaborative research, and provide a model for future international collaborations in nursing. The book concludes with a blueprint for action that nurses can apply to improve the status of nursing education.

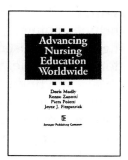

Partial Contents:

Part I: Nursing Education Requirements Worldwide. Global Trends in Nursing Education: A World Health Organization Perspective, *J. Salvage* • Broadening Nursing Boundaries Through Nursing Education and Nursing Education Research, *R. Zanotti*

Part II: Teaching Practices Worldwide. Designing Curriculum to Advance Nursing Science and Practice, *D.M. Modly*

Part III: Issues Important to Nurse Educators Worldwide. Management Education for Nurses in the United States, *S.A. Ryan & C. Conway-Welch* • Computers in Nursing Education, *M. Tallberg* • Re-entry of Students, *D. McGivern*

Part IV: Advancing Research in Nursing Education. Pathways to Implementing Nursing Education Research Globally, *J.J. Fitzpatrick* • A Blueprint for Advancing Nursing Education Research Globally, *Scientific Committee Members*

1995 200pp 0-8261-8650-5 hardcover

536 Broadway, New York, NY 10012-3955 • (212) 431-4370 • Fax (212) 941-7842

S͟P *Springer Publishing Company*

WRITING AND GETTING PUBLISHED
A Primer for Nurses

Barbara Stevens Barnum, RN, PhD, FAAN

This book, by one of nursing's most accomplished authors, is a step-by-step guide to developing professional writing skills and navigating the publication process. It includes pointers on structuring one's writing, avoiding common mistakes, making a term paper or dissertation publishable, writing query letters and book proposals, and finding and working with a publisher. The ability to communicate effectively in writing is an important tool for sharing knowledge and expertise, and for advancing a career. This concise guide demystifies the skills and procedures necessary to make this happen.

Contents:

Part I. Writing the Article • Finding the Right Topic • Writing the Article • Avoiding Common Mistakes • It's a Great Term Paper: Why Don't You Get it Published • Publication Options: Sending Your Article to the Right Journal • What about a Query Letter? • Submitting Articles: Getting the Procedure Right • When Your Article Reaches the Journal

Part II. Writing the Book • How Book Writing Differs from Article Writing • The Edited or Co-authored Book • It's a Great Dissertation, but is it a Book? • Producing the Book Prospectus • Finding and Working with a Publisher

Part III. Special Issues • Writing with Colleagues • Writing from Research • Writing about Work Instruments

Appendices • Appendix A. List of Nursing Journals. • Appendix B. List of Nursing Book Publishers • Appendix C. Additional Writing Resources

1995 216pp   0-8261-8690-4 hardcover

536 Broadway, New York, NY 10012-3955 • (212) 431-4370 • Fax (212) 941-7842